HERBAL ANTIVIRALS

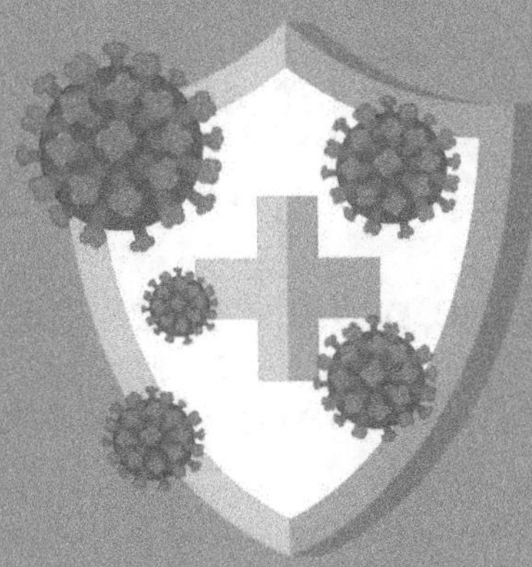

The Complete Step by Step Guide to Choosing and Crafting Effective Herbal Antivirals for Different Ailments

Dr. Diane Reyes

Table of Contents

Introduction: Embracing Herbal Antivirals

Welcome to the realm of herbal antivirals, where ancient wisdom meets modern science in a harmonious symphony of healing. In this introductory chapter, we embark on a journey that transcends conventional medicine, delving into the rich tapestry of nature's pharmacopoeia to unlock the potent secrets of herbal remedies.

For centuries, humanity has turned to the healing embrace of plants to combat viral infections and bolster immune resilience. From the verdant forests of the Amazon to the serene gardens of traditional healers, the lore of herbal medicine has endured as a beacon of hope and vitality in the face of adversity. Now, more than ever, as we navigate the complexities of a rapidly changing world fraught with emerging viral threats, the time has come to rekindle our reverence for nature's bounty.

As a professional doctor and fervent advocate of herbalism, my journey into the realm of herbal antivirals is deeply rooted in personal experience and ancestral wisdom. Inspired by the profound legacy of my grandmother, whose intimate connection with herbs shaped my upbringing in the village of Ikigai, Japan, I have dedicated my life to unravelling the mysteries of botanical medicine.

In this book, I invite you to embark on a transformative odyssey, where each page is imbued with the essence of healing and empowerment. Together, we will explore the multifaceted world of herbal antivirals, from the intricacies of plant chemistry to the art of formulation and preparation. Through a synthesis of ancient knowledge and contemporary research, we will uncover the most potent herbal allies for fortifying immunity, combating viral infections, and nurturing holistic wellness.

But this journey is not merely a quest for knowledge—it is a call to action, a testament to the profound potential that lies within each of us to reclaim our health and vitality. As we navigate the tumultuous waters of the modern world, plagued by the spectre of global pandemics and antibiotic resistance, herbal antivirals offer a beacon of hope, a sanctuary of healing in a world fraught with uncertainty.

So, dear reader, I urge you to embrace the wisdom of herbal antivirals with an open heart and a curious mind. Let us journey together into the verdant realms of nature's pharmacy, where the healing whispers of the earth await to guide us on our path to wellness. With each step we take, may we cultivate a deeper reverence for the interconnected web of life and harness the transformative power of herbal medicine to heal ourselves, our communities, and our planet.

Welcome to the world of herbal antivirals—where healing begins, and possibilities abound. Let us embark on this journey together, as stewards of our health and champions of nature's wisdom.

My Journey into Herbalism: A Personal Introduction

As I pen down these words, I am transported back to the verdant hills of Ikigai, the picturesque village nestled amidst the rolling landscapes of Japan. It is here, amidst the fragrant whispers of herbs and the gentle rustle of leaves, that my journey into herbalism first began—a journey shaped by the timeless wisdom of my grandmother and the profound legacy of my ancestors.

From a tender age, I was enveloped in the embrace of nature's pharmacy, as my grandmother, a revered herbalist in our community, imparted her age-old wisdom with unwavering dedication and boundless love. Every morning, as the first rays of dawn painted the sky in hues of gold, she would lead me through the labyrinthine trails of our ancestral garden, revealing the hidden treasures that lay concealed amidst the emerald foliage.

It was here, amidst the fragrant blossoms of elderflower and the velvety leaves of lemon balm, that I first discovered the transformative power of herbal medicine. With each passing season, my grandmother would share her time-honoured rituals and recipes, weaving tales of healing and resilience that echoed through the annals of time.

One particular memory stands etched in my mind—a memory that serves as a testament to the miraculous potency of herbal antivirals. It was the onset of winter, and a wave of influenza swept through our village with relentless ferocity, leaving many in its wake. As the chilling winds rattled our windows and the whispers of illness echoed through our streets, my grandmother sprung into action, her hands deftly gathering an array of potent herbs from our garden.

With practised precision, she brewed a steaming concoction of elderberry, echinacea, and licorice root—a potent elixir infused with the essence of healing and vitality. As the flames danced in the hearth and the fragrant aroma filled our humble abode, she administered her herbal remedy to those in need, offering solace and relief in the face of adversity.

I watched in awe as the miraculous transformation unfolded before my eyes, witnessing firsthand the profound impact of herbal medicine on the human spirit. It was at that moment that I realised my calling—to carry forth the legacy of my ancestors and champion the healing power of nature's bounty.

Thus, began my journey into herbalism—a journey fueled by a relentless passion for healing and a steadfast commitment to serving others. Armed with the timeless wisdom passed down through generations and fueled by a thirst for knowledge, I embarked on a quest to unravel the mysteries of herbal medicine and harness its transformative potential.

Over the years, my journey has taken me to distant lands and remote corners of the globe, where I have studied under the tutelage of esteemed herbalists and healers.

From the sun-drenched fields of Provence to the mist-shrouded forests of the Amazon, each step of my journey has deepened my understanding of the intricate dance between plants and humanity—a dance woven with threads of healing and hope.

Today, as a professional doctor and herbalist, I stand at the crossroads of tradition and innovation, blending ancient wisdom with modern science to craft holistic solutions for the challenges of our time. Through my herbal apothecary, I have had the privilege of touching the lives of countless individuals, offering solace and support in their moments of need.

But amidst the cacophony of modern life and the relentless march of progress, it is the timeless wisdom of my grandmother that continues to guide my path—a gentle reminder of the profound interconnectedness of all living beings and the sacred bond we share with the natural world.

As I embark on this journey with you, dear reader, I invite you to join me in embracing the healing power of herbalism—a power that transcends the boundaries of time and space, offering solace and sanctuary in a world fraught with uncertainty. Together, let us embark on a transformative odyssey, where each step brings us closer to the vibrant tapestry of life and the boundless possibilities that await in the embrace of nature's bounty.

Welcome to my world of herbalism—a world where healing begins, and miracles unfold with every breath. Together, let us weave a tapestry of wellness and vitality, guided by the timeless wisdom of the earth and the radiant spirit of healing that dwells within us all.

The Evolution of Herbal Antivirals: From Tradition to Modern Science

In the timeless tapestry of human history, the story of herbal antivirals unfolds as a testament to the enduring ingenuity of our ancestors and the boundless potential of nature's pharmacy. From the ancient civilizations of Egypt and China to the vibrant cultures of indigenous peoples around the world, the use of medicinal plants to combat viral infections has been woven into the fabric of our collective consciousness—a legacy of healing that transcends the boundaries of time and space. As I reflect on the evolution of herbal antivirals, I am reminded of the profound legacy of my own ancestors—a legacy steeped in the rich tradition of herbalism and nurtured by the gentle hands of my grandmother, a revered herbalist in our community. It was she who first introduced me to the transformative power of plants, weaving tales of healing and resilience that echoed through the annals of time.

But as we journey through the corridors of history, we witness the inexorable march of progress and the transformative impact of modern science on the field of herbal medicine. In recent decades, advances in technology and research have shed new light on the intricate mechanisms of plant chemistry, unravelling the mysteries of herbal antivirals with unprecedented clarity and precision.

One such milestone in the evolution of herbal antivirals is the discovery of active compounds within medicinal plants—chemical constituents that exhibit potent antiviral properties and hold the key to unlocking nature's healing potential. From the humble elderberry to the majestic echinacea, these botanical treasures have emerged as pillars of resilience in the face of viral adversity, offering solace and support to those in need.

But perhaps the most profound shift in the landscape of herbal antivirals lies in the integration of traditional wisdom with modern science—a synthesis of ancient knowledge and contemporary research that bridges the gap between tradition and innovation. In my own journey as a professional doctor and herbalist, I have witnessed firsthand the transformative power of this synergy, as centuries-old remedies are validated by rigorous scientific inquiry and embraced by a new generation of healers.

One such instance that stands out in my memory is the case of a young woman who sought my aid in her battle against recurrent viral infections. With a history of chronic illness and weakened immunity, she had grown weary of conventional treatments and sought refuge in the gentle embrace of herbal medicine. Drawing upon the timeless wisdom of my grandmother and the latest research in the field, I crafted a bespoke herbal formulation tailored to her unique needs—a potent blend of immune-boosting herbs and antiviral allies.

As she embarked on her journey to wellness, I watched with bated breath as the transformative power of herbal antivirals unfolded before my eyes. With each passing day, her vitality returned, her symptoms abated, and her spirit soared with newfound hope and resilience. It was a testament to the enduring power of nature's bounty and the profound impact of herbal medicine on the human spirit.

In the modern era of global health challenges and emerging viral threats, the need for herbal antivirals has never been greater. From the devastating impact of COVID-19 to the spectre of antibiotic resistance, our world is beset by challenges that demand holistic solutions rooted in the wisdom of nature. As we stand at the crossroads of tradition and innovation, let us embrace the transformative potential of herbal antivirals—a beacon of hope in a world fraught with uncertainty.

Understanding Viral Infections: The Basics and Beyond

Embarking on a journey to unravel the mysteries of viral infections invites us to delve into the depths of a realm where microscopic entities wield profound influence over human health. Unlike bacterial adversaries, these viral invaders cloak themselves in genetic material, instigating a covert onslaught on our cellular fortresses. From the innocuous common cold to the menacing spectre of pandemics like COVID-19, the impact of viral infections reverberates across the tapestry of human existence, shaping the course of history and challenging the boundaries of modern medicine.

To grasp the essence of viral infections is to peer beyond the surface of symptoms and into the intricate dance between host and pathogen—a delicate interplay of molecular machinery and immune response. When a virus infiltrates our cells, it commandeers our biological apparatus with ruthless efficiency, replicating its genetic blueprint and unleashing a cascade of inflammatory reactions. The resulting symptoms, from fever and fatigue to respiratory distress, serve as poignant reminders of the formidable adversaries that lurk within.

As a practitioner of herbal medicine and a steward of ancestral wisdom, my journey into the realm of viral infections has been guided by personal experience and the profound legacy of my forebears. From the time-honoured traditions of herbalism to the frontiers of modern science, I have traversed a vast landscape of knowledge in pursuit of solutions to the complex puzzle of viral afflictions.

Reflecting on this journey, I recall a poignant encounter with a young child grappling with respiratory distress—a poignant reminder of the stakes at hand and the transformative power of herbal remedies. Drawing upon the timeless wisdom of my grandmother and the latest research in the field, I crafted a bespoke herbal formulation tailored to the child's unique needs. With each dose administered, I witnessed the subtle alchemy of nature at work, offering solace and support to a life teetering on the precipice of illness.

Beyond individual cases lies a broader understanding of viral infections as global phenomena, shaped by factors ranging from environmental change to social dynamics. From the rapid spread of infectious diseases in urban centres to the emergence of novel viral strains in the wake of environmental degradation, the challenges we face are as diverse as they are daunting. And yet, amidst the chaos and uncertainty, there is hope—a glimmer of light that emanates from the depths of nature's bounty.

In the pages that follow, we will embark on a journey of discovery and empowerment, guided by the timeless wisdom of the earth and the radiant spirit of healing that dwells within us all. Together, let us explore the multifaceted world of viral infections, from the basics of virology to the latest advancements in herbal antivirals. For in the face of adversity, it is our collective resilience and unwavering determination that will carry us through, offering solace and support in our quest for health and well-being.

Chapter 1: Building Your Herbal Arsenal

Welcome to the gateway of herbal wisdom, where the keys to holistic wellness and vitality await at your fingertips. In this foundational chapter, we embark on a journey of discovery and empowerment, as we lay the groundwork for building your very own herbal arsenal—a treasure trove of botanical allies to support your health and well-being in the face of life's myriad challenges.

I have long been captivated by the transformative power of plants to heal and nurture the body, mind, and spirit. From the verdant hills of Ikigai to the bustling streets of modern cities, the legacy of herbalism has endured as a beacon of hope and resilience in the face of adversity.

One of the first steps in building your herbal arsenal is to cultivate a deep reverence for the plants themselves—a profound appreciation for their resilience, diversity, and healing potential. Whether it be the delicate petals of chamomile or the sturdy leaves of echinacea, each plant possesses a unique constellation of compounds and qualities that make it a valuable ally in the quest for wellness.

Beyond mere admiration lies the practical art of herbal preparation—an essential skill that empowers you to harness the healing power of plants in your own life. From simple teas and tinctures to more complex formulations and extracts, the possibilities are endless, limited only by your imagination and creativity.

In my own journey as a healer and herbalist, I have witnessed the transformative impact of herbal remedies on countless individuals grappling with viral infections and other health challenges. From the soothing embrace of elderberry syrup to the potent antimicrobial properties of garlic, each herbal ally offers a unique pathway to wellness, tailored to the individual needs of the body and spirit.

But perhaps the most profound aspect of building your herbal arsenal lies in the journey itself—a journey of self-discovery and empowerment that transcends the boundaries of illness and adversity. As you delve deeper into the world of herbal medicine, you will cultivate a deeper connection with the natural world and a profound sense of agency over your own health and well-being.

In the chapters that follow, we will explore a myriad of herbal allies and formulations, from immune-boosting elixirs to soothing balms for the soul. Together, let us embark on a journey of exploration and enlightenment, guided by the timeless wisdom of the earth and the radiant spirit of healing that dwells within us all. For in the gentle embrace of nature's bounty lies the key to unlocking a lifetime of health, vitality, and holistic wellness.

Selecting and Sourcing High-Quality Herbs

As we embark on the journey of building our herbal arsenal, one of the most critical steps is the careful selection and sourcing of high-quality herbs. In this chapter, we delve into the intricacies of identifying and procuring herbs that embody the essence of purity, potency, and efficacy—a task that requires both discernment and diligence.

Throughout my years as a practitioner of herbal medicine, I have come to appreciate the profound impact that the quality of herbs can have on the effectiveness of herbal remedies. From the lush forests of Japan to the verdant fields of my own herbal garden, I have witnessed firsthand the transformative power of herbs sourced with care and intention.

One of the first considerations when selecting herbs is their origin and growing conditions. Ideally, herbs should be grown in environments free from pesticides, herbicides, and other harmful chemicals, ensuring that they retain their natural vitality and therapeutic properties. Whether harvested from wild landscapes or cultivated with care, the purity of the growing environment plays a pivotal role in determining the quality of the final product.

In my own practice, I have cultivated a deep reverence for the plants themselves, often sourcing herbs from local growers and wildcrafters who share my commitment to sustainability and stewardship of the land. By forging connections with these dedicated individuals, I am able to ensure that the herbs I use are not only of the highest quality but also imbued with a sense of integrity and respect for the natural world.

Another important consideration when selecting herbs is their method of processing and preparation. Herbs that are harvested at the peak of their potency and processed with care retain the full spectrum of their therapeutic compounds, ensuring maximum efficacy and bioavailability. Whether dried for teas and tinctures or extracted into potent herbal remedies, the manner in which herbs are prepared can greatly influence their healing potential.

In my own herbal apothecary, I take great care to process herbs using methods that preserve their natural integrity and vitality. From handcrafting small-batch tinctures to sun-drying herbs for teas and infusions, each step of the process is infused with intention and reverence for the plants themselves. By honouring the wisdom of traditional herbal preparations while embracing modern innovations, I am able to offer my clients herbal remedies of the highest quality and efficacy.

Ultimately, the selection and sourcing of high-quality herbs is a journey of discovery and connection—a journey that invites us to cultivate a deeper relationship with the natural world and the healing power of plants. By choosing herbs that are grown and processed with care, we honour not only the wisdom of ancient traditions but also the innate intelligence of the earth itself.

Identifying High-Quality Herbs:

Research and Education: Begin by educating yourself about the herbs you wish to procure. Understand their botanical characteristics, growing conditions, and potential variations in quality.

Appearance and Aroma: High-quality herbs often exhibit vibrant colours, distinct aromas, and intact, unblemished leaves or flowers. Look for herbs that appear fresh and vibrant, with no signs of mould or discoloration.

Texture and Consistency: The texture of dried herbs should be neither excessively dry nor overly moist. They should crumble easily between your fingers without feeling brittle or powdery.

Purity and Authenticity: Ensure that the herbs you purchase are free from adulterants, fillers, or contaminants. Look for reputable suppliers who prioritise transparency and quality assurance.

Sourcing High-Quality Herbs:

Local Growers and Wildcrafters: Build relationships with local growers, farmers, and wildcrafters who cultivate or harvest herbs with care and integrity. Visit farmers' markets, herbal conferences, or community gardens to connect with like-minded individuals.

Certifications and Standards: Look for herbs that are certified organic or grown using sustainable practices. Certifications such as USDA Organic or Fair Wild provide assurance of ethical sourcing and environmental stewardship.

Online Suppliers: While online suppliers offer convenience and access to a wide range of herbs, exercise caution and research the reputation and credibility of the supplier.

Look for reviews, certifications, and transparent sourcing practices.

Wildcrafting: If harvesting wild herbs, do so responsibly and ethically. Obtain necessary permits, respect local regulations, and avoid overharvesting or damaging delicate ecosystems.

By following these guidelines, you can ensure that the herbs you select and source for your herbal arsenal are of the highest quality, potency, and efficacy. Remember that each herb carries its own unique energy and healing properties, and by choosing with intention and care, you honour the wisdom of nature and empower yourself on your journey of herbal wellness.

Herbal Preparation Methods: Infusions, Decoctions, Tinctures, and More

In our quest to build a robust herbal arsenal, mastering the art of herbal preparation methods is essential. From the soothing embrace of herbal teas to the potent extracts of tinctures, each method offers a unique pathway to harnessing the healing power of plants. In this chapter, we explore the various techniques for preparing and utilising herbs, empowering you to craft potent remedies tailored to your specific needs.

Throughout my journey as a healer and herbalist, I have witnessed the profound impact that herbal preparation methods can have on the effectiveness and potency of herbal remedies. Whether brewing a cup of chamomile tea to soothe the nerves or concocting a tincture of echinacea to bolster the immune system, the manner in which herbs are prepared can greatly influence their therapeutic properties.

Infusions:

Infusions, also known as herbal teas, are perhaps the most familiar and accessible method of herbal preparation. By steeping herbs in hot water, we extract their medicinal compounds and create a soothing and nourishing beverage. To prepare an infusion, simply pour hot water over the desired herbs, cover, and allow to steep for 5-10 minutes. Strain and enjoy as desired.

Decoctions:

Decoctions are another traditional method of herbal preparation, particularly suited for tougher plant materials such as roots, barks, and seeds. To prepare a decoction, simmer the desired herbs in water for 20-30 minutes, allowing the heat to extract their medicinal properties. Strain and consume the resulting liquid as a potent herbal remedy.

Tinctures:

Tinctures are concentrated herbal extracts made by macerating herbs in alcohol or vinegar. This method effectively extracts the active constituents of the herbs, creating a potent and shelf-stable remedy. To prepare a tincture, fill a glass jar with chopped herbs and cover with alcohol or vinegar. Allow to steep for several weeks, shaking the jar regularly to ensure thorough extraction. Strain and bottle the resulting liquid for long-term storage and use.

Poultices and Compresses:

Poultices and compresses are external applications of herbs, used to soothe inflammation, relieve pain, and promote healing. To prepare a poultice, simply crush fresh or dried herbs and apply directly to the affected area, covering with a clean cloth or bandage. Compresses involve soaking a cloth in a strong herbal infusion or decoction and applying it to the skin as needed.

Syrups and Elixirs:

Syrups and elixirs offer a delicious and convenient way to consume herbal remedies, particularly for children or those with sensitive palates. To prepare a syrup, simmer herbs in water to create a strong infusion, then strain and sweeten with honey or sugar. Elixirs involve combining herbal extracts with honey, glycerin, or other sweeteners for a flavorful and potent remedy.

By mastering these herbal preparation methods, you can unlock the full potential of nature's pharmacy and create customised remedies tailored to your unique needs and preferences. Whether sipping a soothing herbal tea or applying a healing poultice, let the wisdom of the plants guide you on your journey to health and vitality.

Essential Tools for Herbal Medicine Making

As we embark on the journey of building our herbal arsenal, it is essential to equip ourselves with the proper tools and equipment for herbal medicine making. From measuring and mixing to straining and bottling, having the right tools at our disposal ensures that we can craft potent and effective remedies with precision and ease. In this chapter, we explore the essential tools necessary for herbal medicine making, empowering you to unleash the full potential of nature's healing bounty.

Throughout my years of practice as a healer and herbalist, I have come to appreciate the importance of having a well-stocked herbal apothecary equipped with high-quality tools and equipment. Whether preparing tinctures, salves, or teas, having the right tools on hand allows me to create remedies that are not only potent and effective but also infused with intention and care.

Measuring Tools:

Accurate measurement is crucial in herbal medicine making to ensure consistency and efficacy. Essential measuring tools include:

Measuring Spoons and Cups: For precise measurement of herbs, liquids, and other ingredients.

Graduated Cylinders: Ideal for measuring liquids, particularly when preparing tinctures and extracts.

Digital Scale: Provides accurate measurement of herbs and other ingredients by weight, ensuring precise formulation.

Mixing and Straining Equipment:

Proper mixing and straining are essential steps in herbal medicine making to extract and blend the medicinal properties of herbs. Essential equipment includes:

Glass Mixing Bowls: Non-reactive and easy to clean, glass bowls are ideal for mixing herbal preparations.

Stainless Steel Strainers: For straining herbal infusions, decoctions, and tinctures, ensuring a smooth and debris-free final product.

Cheesecloth or Muslin Bags: Used for straining herbs and extracting liquids, providing a fine filtration to remove particles and sediment.

Storage and Bottling Supplies:

Once herbal remedies are prepared, proper storage is essential to maintain their potency and freshness. Essential storage and bottling supplies include:

Glass Jars and Bottles: Dark-coloured glass jars and bottles protect herbal remedies from light and air, preserving their potency and shelf life.

Labels and Markers: Essential for labelling herbal preparations with ingredients, date of preparation, and dosage instructions, ensuring clarity and safety.

Pipettes and Droppers: For dispensing precise doses of liquid herbal remedies, ensuring accurate administration and dosage.

Miscellaneous Tools:

In addition to the essential tools mentioned above, there are several miscellaneous tools that can enhance the herbal medicine making process, including:

Herb Grinder or Mortar and Pestle: For grinding dried herbs into powder or breaking down fresh herbs for extraction.

Double Boiler: Ideal for gentle heating and melting of ingredients, particularly when preparing salves and balms.

Funnel: Facilitates easy and mess-free transfer of herbal preparations into bottles and jars.

By equipping yourself with these essential tools for herbal medicine making, you can embark on your journey with confidence, knowing that you have everything you need to create potent and effective remedies. Whether concocting a soothing herbal tea or formulating a healing salve, let these tools be your trusted companions on the path to wellness and vitality.

Chapter 2: Key Herbal Antivirals and Their Properties

In delving deeper into the realm of herbal antivirals, we uncover a treasure trove of botanical allies that possess potent antiviral properties. As we journey through this chapter, we will explore the diverse array of herbs renowned for their ability to combat viral infections and bolster the body's innate defences against pathogens. Drawing upon my extensive experience as a healer and herbalist, I will guide you through the properties and uses of these key herbal antivirals, empowering you to harness their healing potential for yourself and your loved ones.

Exploring Nature's Pharmacy:

Nature has long been our greatest ally in the fight against viral infections, offering a bounty of medicinal plants with powerful antiviral properties. From the verdant forests of Japan to the sun-drenched fields of the Mediterranean, cultures around the world have relied on herbal remedies to combat viral illnesses for centuries. In my own practice, I have witnessed the remarkable efficacy of these botanical medicines in treating a wide range of viral infections, from the common cold to more serious illnesses.

The Power of Plant Medicine:

At the heart of herbal antivirals lies the potent bioactive compounds found within the plants themselves. These compounds, such as polyphenols, flavonoids, and terpenes, possess powerful antiviral, anti-inflammatory, and immune-modulating properties that can help fortify the body's defences against viral invaders. By harnessing the healing power of these plant constituents, we can support the body's natural ability to fight off infections and promote overall wellness.

Key Herbal Antivirals:

Among the vast array of medicinal plants, several stand out as potent herbal antivirals with well-documented efficacy in combating viral infections. From the immune-boosting echinacea to the antimicrobial garlic, each herb offers a unique set of properties that make it a valuable addition to our herbal arsenal. Throughout this chapter, we will explore the properties and uses of these key herbal antivirals, including how to prepare and administer them for optimal efficacy.

Empowering Yourself with Knowledge:

As we journey through this chapter, my hope is to empower you with the knowledge and tools you need to take control of your health and well-being. By understanding the properties and uses of key herbal antivirals, you can make informed decisions about how best to support your body's immune system and protect yourself against viral infections. Whether brewing a cup of immune-boosting tea or formulating a potent tincture, let the wisdom of nature be your guide on the path to vibrant health and vitality.

In the next sections, we will delve into the specifics of each herbal antiviral, exploring their unique properties, preparation methods, and therapeutic uses. By immersing ourselves in the rich tapestry of plant medicine, we can unlock the full potential of herbal antivirals and harness the healing power of nature to safeguard our health and well-being.

Exploring Nature's Pharmacy: Profiles of Powerful Antiviral Plants

In the realm of herbal medicine, the intricate dance between humanity and nature unfolds with each discovery of a potent botanical ally. As a dedicated herbalist, I have traversed this fertile landscape, guided by ancestral wisdom and fueled by a passion for healing. Join me now as we embark on a journey through nature's pharmacy, where we shall unveil the profiles of several remarkable antiviral plants, each offering its unique gifts to support our well-being and resilience.

Echinacea (Echinacea purpurea):

Imagine standing amidst a field of vibrant purple echinacea blooms, their petals dancing in the gentle breeze, their roots firmly anchored in the earth. It was here, amidst this breathtaking display of nature's splendour, that I first encountered the profound healing potential of echinacea. Drawing upon centuries of traditional use and modern scientific research, echinacea has emerged as a formidable ally in the fight against viral infections. Its ability to stimulate the immune system and reduce the severity and duration of colds and flu is nothing short of remarkable. From tinctures to teas, echinacea stands as a cornerstone in the herbal arsenal, offering solace and support to those in need.

Garlic (Allium sativum):

Step into the warmth of a rustic kitchen, where the pungent aroma of garlic fills the air, infusing every dish with its unmistakable flavour and healing properties. From ancient civilizations to modern-day herbalists, garlic has held a revered place in the pantheon of medicinal plants. Rich in allicin and other bioactive compounds, garlic exhibits potent antiviral properties, making it a valuable ally in the fight against respiratory infections and other viral maladies. Whether consumed raw, cooked, or in supplement form, garlic stands as a testament to nature's power to heal and protect.

Elderberry (Sambucus nigra):

Picture a sprawling elderberry bush, laden with clusters of dark purple berries glistening in the sunlight like precious jewels. For generations, elderberry has been cherished for its immune-boosting properties and ability to ward off colds, flu, and other viral infections. Rich in flavonoids and antioxidants, elderberry syrup has become a staple in many households during the cold winter months, offering both comfort and protection against seasonal ailments. From soothing sore throats to reducing inflammation, elderberry remains a cherished ally in the herbalist's toolkit.

Licorice Root (Glycyrrhiza glabra):

Venture into the bustling aisles of a vibrant market, where bundles of licorice root beckon with their earthy aroma and myriad healing properties. Revered for centuries in traditional medicine systems around the world, licorice root boasts potent antiviral and immune-modulating effects. Its active compound, glycyrrhizin, has been shown to inhibit the replication of viruses and reduce the severity of symptoms associated with respiratory infections. Whether brewed into a tea or incorporated into herbal formulations, licorice root offers a sweet and soothing remedy for those in need of healing.

Ginger (Zingiber officinale):

Close your eyes and envision a steaming cup of ginger tea, its fiery warmth spreading comfort and vitality throughout your body. With its invigorating aroma and spicy flavour, ginger has long been revered for its ability to alleviate nausea, aid digestion, and boost the immune system. Rich in bioactive compounds such as gingerol and shogaol, ginger exhibits potent antiviral properties, making it a valuable ally in the fight against colds, flu, and other viral infections. Whether grated fresh into tea or infused into syrups and tinctures, ginger stands as a testament to the power of nature to nurture and heal.

As we traverse the verdant landscapes of nature's pharmacy, let us embrace the wisdom of the ages while remaining open to the insights of modern science. With each step forward, may we deepen our understanding of these potent botanical allies and harness their healing gifts to cultivate resilience, vitality, and well-being.

From the Garden to Your Medicine Cabinet: Growing and Harvesting Herbs at Home

Welcome to the verdant realm of your own herbal sanctuary, where the gentle rustle of leaves and the vibrant hues of blossoms beckon you into a world of healing and vitality. As a steward of herbal wisdom and a custodian of nature's bounty, I am delighted to guide you on a journey from seed to remedy, where the act of growing and harvesting herbs at home becomes a sacred ritual of connection and empowerment.

Cultivating Your Herbal Oasis:

Imagine the sun-kissed tranquillity of your own garden, where rows of fragrant herbs sway in harmony with the rhythm of the earth. From the humble beginnings of a single seed to the lush abundance of a thriving herbal oasis, the act of cultivation becomes a labour of love and a testament to the resilience of nature's wisdom. Whether nestled in raised beds, window boxes, or sprawling across a sunlit patch of earth, your herbal garden becomes a sanctuary of healing, offering solace and sustenance to both body and soul.

Tending to the Sacred Cycle:

As the seasons ebb and flow, so too does the sacred cycle of growth and renewal within your herbal garden. With each passing month, you witness the delicate dance of life unfolding before your eyes, from the tender emergence of seedlings in spring to the bountiful harvests of summer's abundance. With gentle hands and a heart attuned to the rhythms of nature, you nurture your herbal allies, fostering their growth with care and reverence. Through the ancient art of herbalism, you become a co-creator in the unfolding tapestry of life, honouring the interconnectedness of all beings and the wisdom of the natural world.

Harvesting the Fruits of Your Labor:

As the sun reaches its zenith and the air hums with the symphony of nature's bounty, the time has come to gather the fruits of your labour and bring them home to your medicine cabinet. With a sense of gratitude and reverence, you carefully harvest your herbs, mindful of the delicate balance between giving and receiving. From vibrant leaves to fragrant blossoms, each plant offers its unique gifts, imbued with the healing essence of the earth. With each snip of the shears and each gentle touch, you honour the ancient lineage of herbal wisdom passed down through generations, weaving your own story into the rich tapestry of herbal lore.

Crafting Your Herbal Remedies:

With an abundance of freshly harvested herbs at your fingertips, the time has come to craft your own herbal remedies, transforming nature's gifts into potent elixirs of healing and vitality. From soothing salves to invigorating tinctures, the possibilities are as endless as the boundless creativity of the human spirit. With each infusion and each decoction, you infuse your remedies with the essence of your own intentions, imbuing them with the healing power of love and compassion. As you stand before your medicine cabinet, surrounded by jars of herbal treasures, you are reminded of the profound connection between earth and body, heart and soul.

Conclusion:

In the garden of herbal wisdom, the journey from seed to remedy is a sacred pilgrimage of connection and transformation. Through the act of growing and harvesting herbs at home, we honour the timeless rhythms of nature and cultivate a deeper relationship with the healing power of the earth. As we tend to our herbal allies with care and reverence, we become stewards of a living legacy, preserving the ancient wisdom of herbalism for generations to come. So let us embrace the gentle whispers of the wind and the steady pulse of the earth, for in the garden of our hearts, the seeds of healing are forever sown.

Unlocking the Antiviral Potential: Understanding Active Compounds

As a practitioner deeply immersed in the world of herbalism, I've come to appreciate the intricate complexities of plant compounds and their remarkable antiviral properties. In this chapter, we embark on a journey to explore the hidden treasures within nature's pharmacy, delving into the fascinating realm of active compounds that hold the key to unlocking the antiviral potential of plants.

At the heart of herbal medicine lies a profound understanding of the bioactive molecules synthesised by plants, known as active compounds. These compounds are the chemical constituents responsible for the therapeutic effects observed in herbal remedies. Understanding their properties, mechanisms of action, and interactions is essential for harnessing their full healing potential.

One of the primary classes of active compounds found in antiviral herbs is polyphenols. These potent antioxidants exhibit a wide range of antiviral activities, including inhibiting viral replication, modulating immune responses, and reducing inflammation. Examples of polyphenols with proven antiviral properties include flavonoids, phenolic acids, and tannins, which can be found in plants such as elderberry, licorice root, and green tea.

Terpenoids represent another crucial group of active compounds renowned for their antiviral effects. These aromatic molecules, abundant in essential oils, possess diverse biological activities, including antiviral, antimicrobial, and anti-inflammatory properties. Menthol from peppermint, eugenol from cloves, and limonene from citrus fruits are just a few examples of terpenoids known for their potent antiviral actions.

Additionally, alkaloids, glycosides, and polysaccharides are among the many other classes of active compounds found in antiviral herbs, each contributing unique therapeutic benefits. Alkaloids like berberine in goldenseal exhibit broad-spectrum antiviral activity, while polysaccharides from medicinal mushrooms such as reishi enhance immune function, aiding in viral defence.

Furthermore, it's essential to recognize the synergistic interactions between these active compounds within herbal formulations. The holistic approach of herbal medicine acknowledges that the combined action of multiple compounds often yields greater therapeutic effects than any single constituent alone—a concept known as the entourage effect.

As we delve deeper into the realm of active compounds, we gain a profound appreciation for the intricate tapestry of nature's pharmacopoeia. By understanding the diverse array of bioactive molecules present in antiviral herbs, we empower ourselves to harness their full therapeutic potential in combating viral infections and promoting holistic wellness.

Chapter 3: Crafting Effective Herbal Formulations

Herbal Combinations for Enhanced Antiviral Activity

Throughout history, plants have played a vital role in human health and healing. Long before the advent of modern medicine, our ancestors relied on the natural remedies derived from herbs and plants to treat various ailments, including viral infections. While many conventional antiviral drugs have been developed, the field of herbal medicine continues to offer promising alternatives and complementary approaches. One particularly intriguing concept is the use of herbal combinations, where multiple herbs are carefully blended to achieve enhanced therapeutic effects. The rationale behind this approach lies in the synergistic interactions that can occur when different plants with distinct phytochemical profiles are combined. By harnessing the collective power of these natural compounds, herbal combinations may exhibit potent antiviral activities that surpass the capabilities of individual herbs.

The Synergy of Nature's Bounty

Herbs are rich sources of a wide range of bioactive compounds, such as flavonoids, alkaloids, terpenoids, and polyphenols, among many others. These phytochemicals possess diverse biological properties, including antiviral, anti-inflammatory, and immunomodulatory effects. When combined strategically, these compounds can work together in a synergistic manner, amplifying their individual effects and targeting multiple pathways involved in viral infections.

One of the primary mechanisms by which herbal combinations exert their antiviral effects is by inhibiting viral entry and attachment to host cells. Certain herbs contain compounds that can bind to viral surface proteins or cellular receptors, effectively blocking the virus from gaining access to the host cells. For instance, the combination of elderberry, echinacea, and goldenseal has been studied for its potential to disrupt the entry of influenza viruses into cells.

Another mechanism involves the disruption of viral replication. Once a virus has successfully entered a host cell, it hijacks the cell's machinery to produce more copies of itself. However, some herbal compounds can interfere with this process by inhibiting viral enzymes or disrupting the synthesis of viral proteins and nucleic acids. The combination of licorice, isatis, and forsythia, for example, has been explored for its ability to impede the replication of various viruses, including SARS-CoV-2, the virus responsible for COVID-19.

Additionally, herbal combinations can modulate the immune system, enhancing the body's natural defences against viral infections. Certain herbs possess immunomodulatory properties that can stimulate the production of cytokines, activate immune cells, and regulate inflammatory responses. The combination of garlic, ginger, and turmeric, for instance, has been studied for its potential to support a balanced immune response and reduce inflammation associated with viral infections.

Promising Herbal Combinations

While numerous herbal combinations have been explored for their antiviral properties, some particularly promising examples include:

Elderberry, Echinacea, and Goldenseal: This trio has been traditionally used to treat respiratory infections and has demonstrated potential antiviral activity against influenza and other respiratory viruses.

Licorice, Isatis, and Forsythia: Common ingredients in traditional Chinese medicine formulations, these herbs have shown antiviral effects against various viruses, including SARS-CoV-2, through mechanisms such as inhibiting viral entry and replication.

Garlic, Ginger, and Turmeric: Well-known for their anti-inflammatory and antioxidant properties, this combination has exhibited potential antiviral effects against a range of viruses, likely due to their ability to modulate the immune response.

Green Tea, Pomegranate, and Resveratrol: Rich in polyphenolic compounds, this combination has been studied for its antiviral activity against influenza, HIV, and hepatitis viruses, potentially by inhibiting viral entry and replication.

It's important to note that while these herbal combinations hold promise, their efficacy and safety must be thoroughly evaluated through rigorous clinical studies. Additionally, proper formulation, dosing, and quality control are crucial to ensure consistent and reliable results.

Embracing Nature's Wisdom

The exploration of herbal combinations for antiviral activity represents a fascinating intersection of traditional knowledge and modern scientific inquiry. By harnessing the synergistic effects of nature's bounty, we may unlock new avenues for combating viral infections and supporting overall health and well-being.

However, it is essential to approach herbal remedies with caution and seek guidance from qualified healthcare professionals. Potential herb-drug interactions, contraindications, and side effects must be carefully considered. Furthermore, the quality and standardisation of herbal products should be ensured to maintain consistency and safety.

As we continue to navigate the challenges posed by emerging and evolving viral threats, the integration of herbal medicine with conventional antiviral therapies may offer a promising complementary approach. By embracing the wisdom of nature and fostering collaboration between traditional and modern medical practices, we can potentially enhance our arsenal against viral infections and promote holistic healing.

The pursuit of knowledge in the realm of herbal combinations for antiviral activity is an ongoing journey, one that requires dedication, scientific rigour, and an open mind. As we delve deeper into this fascinating field, we may uncover nature's secrets and harness the power of plant synergy for the betterment of human health.

Herbal Synergy: Understanding How Plants Work Together

The ancient practice of using herbs for medicinal purposes has been a foundation of traditional healing systems around the world. Over centuries, humans have harnessed the power of plants to treat various ailments and promote overall well-being. However, the true potential of herbal medicine lies not only in the individual properties of each plant but also in the synergistic interactions that occur when multiple herbs are combined.

Herbal synergy, also known as polyherbal formulation or herbal combination, is the concept of blending different herbs to achieve a more potent therapeutic effect than any single herb could provide alone. This synergistic approach has been an integral part of many traditional medicine systems, such as Ayurveda, Traditional Chinese Medicine (TCM), and Western herbal medicine.

The Science Behind Herbal Synergy

Plants are complex organisms that produce a vast array of phytochemicals, including flavonoids, alkaloids, terpenes, and polyphenols, among many others. These compounds are responsible for the medicinal properties of herbs and interact with various biological systems in the human body. When different herbs are combined, their phytochemicals can work together in a synergistic manner, amplifying their individual effects and targeting multiple pathways simultaneously.

There are several mechanisms by which herbal synergy can occur:

Additive Effect: In this scenario, the combined effects of multiple herbs are simply the sum of their individual effects. Each herb contributes its unique properties, and the overall effect is an accumulation of these properties.

Synergistic Effect: This occurs when the combination of herbs produces an effect that is greater than the sum of their individual effects. The phytochemicals in different herbs can interact in a way that enhances their overall potency, resulting in a more profound therapeutic impact.

Complementary Effect: Certain herbs may have complementary actions that support or enhance the effects of other herbs in the combination. For example, one herb may target a specific pathway, while another herb addresses a different aspect of the same condition, resulting in a more comprehensive therapeutic approach.

Counteractive Effect: In some cases, herbs can counteract or mitigate the potential side effects or toxicities of other herbs in the combination. This can improve the overall safety and tolerability of the herbal formulation.

Promising Herbal Combinations

Throughout history, various traditional medicine systems have developed numerous herbal combinations that leverage the power of synergy. Here are a few examples of promising herbal combinations and their potential applications:

Triphala: A renowned Ayurvedic formulation comprising three fruits – Amalaki (Emblica officinalis), Bibhitaki (Terminalia bellirica), and Haritaki (Terminalia chebula). This combination is widely used for digestive health, detoxification, and as a rejuvenating tonic.

Kan Jang: A Traditional Chinese Medicine formula consisting of Glycyrrhiza glabra (licorice root), Ephedra sinica (ephedra), and Zingiber officinale (ginger). It has been used to treat respiratory conditions, such as asthma and bronchitis, due to its anti-inflammatory and bronchodilatory effects.

Essiac Tea: A Native American herbal blend composed of burdock root, slippery elm bark, sheep sorrel, and Turkish rhubarb root. This combination has been traditionally used for its potential anticancer and immune-boosting properties.

St. John's Wort and Black Cohosh: A combination of St. John's Wort (Hypericum perforatum) and Black Cohosh (Actaea racemosa) has been studied for its potential in alleviating menopausal symptoms, such as hot flashes and mood disturbances, due to their complementary actions.

Garlic and Ginger: A popular combination in many culinary traditions, garlic (Allium sativum) and ginger (Zingiber officinale) have been used for their anti-inflammatory, antimicrobial, and immune-boosting properties, particularly in the treatment of respiratory infections and digestive issues.

While these examples illustrate the potential benefits of herbal synergy, it is crucial to note that the efficacy and safety of herbal combinations should be thoroughly evaluated through rigorous scientific research. Quality control, standardisation, and proper dosing are essential to ensure consistent and reliable results.

The Future of Herbal Synergy

As the field of herbal medicine continues to evolve, the concept of herbal synergy presents exciting opportunities for advancing our understanding of plant-based therapeutics. By combining traditional knowledge with modern scientific techniques, researchers can unravel the intricate interactions between phytochemicals and their effects on various biological systems.

One promising area of research is the exploration of novel herbal combinations tailored to specific health conditions or therapeutic targets. Through systematic screening and evaluation, researchers can identify synergistic combinations that exhibit enhanced potency, improved safety profiles, or unique mechanisms of action.

Additionally, the integration of herbal synergy with conventional medical approaches holds potential for developing complementary and integrative therapies. By combining the strengths of both traditional and modern medicine, healthcare professionals may be able to provide more comprehensive and holistic treatment options for their patients.

Furthermore, advances in analytical techniques, such as metabolomics and network pharmacology, can shed light on the intricate interactions between phytochemicals and their effects on biological pathways. These insights can inform the development of more effective and targeted herbal formulations.

Conclusion

Herbal synergy represents a fascinating intersection of traditional wisdom and modern scientific inquiry. By understanding how plants work together, we can unlock the full potential of herbal medicine and develop more effective and holistic therapeutic approaches. As we continue to explore the synergistic interactions between herbs, we may uncover new avenues for promoting better health and well-being.

However, it is essential to approach herbal medicine with caution and seek guidance from qualified healthcare professionals. Quality control, standardisation, and proper dosing are crucial to ensure safe and effective use of herbal combinations. By fostering collaboration between traditional healing systems and modern medical practices, we can harness the power of herbal synergy while prioritising patient safety and evidence-based approaches.

Dosage Guidelines and Administration Techniques

In the realm of herbal medicine, antiviral herbs have gained significant attention for their potential in combating viral infections. While these natural remedies offer promising therapeutic benefits, it is crucial to understand the appropriate dosage guidelines and administration techniques to ensure their safe and effective use.

Dosage Guidelines for Herbal Antivirals

Determining the correct dosage for herbal antivirals involves considering several factors, including the specific herb, the condition being treated, and the individual characteristics of the patient.

Herb-specific dosages:

Each herb has its own unique composition of active compounds and, consequently, its own recommended dosage range.

Dosages are typically expressed in dry weight measurements, such as milligrams (mg) or grams (g), for standardised extracts or dried herb preparations.

Condition and severity:

The dosage may vary depending on the type of viral infection and its severity.
More severe or acute infections may require higher dosages to achieve the desired antiviral effects.

Patient factors:

Age: Dosages may need to be adjusted for paediatric and geriatric populations due to differences in metabolism and potential sensitivity.
Weight: Some herbal dosages are based on the patient's body weight, particularly for children.
Pregnancy and lactation: Certain herbs may have contraindications or require

dosage adjustments during these physiological states.

Duration of use:

Acute viral infections may require higher dosages for a shorter duration, while chronic conditions may necessitate lower dosages over an extended period.
It is essential to consult reliable sources, such as reputable herbal monographs, clinical studies, or experienced herbalists, to determine the appropriate dosage range for each specific herb and clinical situation.

Administration Techniques for Herbal Antivirals

The administration technique for herbal antivirals can vary depending on the form of the herbal preparation and the desired route of administration. Common administration techniques include:

Oral administration:

Teas and infusions: Steeping dried herbs in hot water and consuming the resulting tea is a common method of administration. Proper brewing techniques and steeping times should be followed.

Capsules and tablets: Encapsulated or tableted forms of herbal extracts or powders can be swallowed with water or other liquids.

Tinctures and liquid extracts: These concentrated liquid preparations are typically taken by the dropperful, mixed with water or juice.

Topical application:

Ointments, creams, and salves: For certain viral infections affecting the skin or mucous membranes, herbal preparations can be applied topically. Proper application techniques and adherence to instructions are crucial.

Inhalation:

Steam inhalation: Some antiviral herbs can be added to steaming water for inhalation, potentially beneficial for respiratory viral infections. Appropriate precautions should be taken to avoid burns or irritation.

Parenteral administration:

Injectable forms: While less common, some herbal extracts or isolated compounds may be available in injectable forms for specific clinical applications, requiring proper aseptic technique and administration by qualified healthcare professionals.

Factors Influencing Dosage and Administration

Several factors can influence the dosage and administration of herbal antivirals, including:

Herb-drug interactions:

Certain herbs may interact with prescription medications, potentially altering their efficacy or increasing the risk of adverse effects. Consulting healthcare providers is essential to avoid potential interactions.

Quality and standardisation:

The quality and standardisation of herbal products can vary significantly, impacting their potency and safety. Choosing reputable brands and consulting healthcare professionals is recommended.

Comorbidities and concomitant conditions:

Patients with underlying medical conditions, such as liver or kidney dysfunction, may require dosage adjustments or specific administration considerations.

Cultural and personal preferences:

Respecting cultural beliefs, personal preferences, and involving patients in decision-making can improve adherence and therapeutic outcomes.

Patient education and adherence:

Providing clear instructions, addressing concerns, and promoting patient engagement can improve adherence to dosage and administration guidelines for herbal antivirals.

Importance of Proper Dosage and Administration

Adhering to appropriate dosage guidelines and proper administration techniques is crucial for ensuring the safety and efficacy of herbal antivirals. Incorrect dosing or improper administration can lead to adverse effects, treatment failures, or potentially life-threatening consequences.

By following evidence-based dosage guidelines and utilising appropriate administration techniques, healthcare professionals and patients can optimise the therapeutic benefits of herbal antivirals while minimising potential risks and adverse events.

It is important to note that while herbal remedies are often perceived as natural and safe, they can still interact with medications and potentially cause adverse effects if not used properly. Consulting with qualified healthcare professionals, such as herbalists, naturopathic doctors, or integrative medicine practitioners, is strongly recommended to ensure the safe and effective use of herbal antivirals.

Conclusion

Dosage guidelines and administration techniques play a crucial role in the safe and effective use of herbal antivirals. By carefully considering factors such as the specific herb, condition being treated, patient characteristics, and potential interactions, healthcare professionals and patients can maximise the therapeutic benefits while minimising potential risks.

Continuous education, staying updated with current research and guidelines, and fostering open communication between healthcare providers and patients are essential steps in achieving successful outcomes with herbal antiviral treatments. Additionally, promoting quality control and standardisation in the herbal product industry is vital to ensure consistent and reliable results.

As the interest in natural remedies continues to grow, it is essential to approach herbal antivirals with a balanced and evidence-based perspective, combining traditional knowledge with modern scientific understanding to ensure their safe and effective integration into healthcare practices.

Chapter 4: Addressing Specific Viral Infections

Targeting Respiratory Viruses: Herbs for Colds, Flu, and Beyond

Respiratory viral infections, such as the common cold, influenza, and respiratory syncytial virus (RSV), are among the most prevalent and burdensome illnesses worldwide. While conventional antiviral medications are available, many people seek natural alternatives, particularly herbal remedies, to alleviate symptoms and support their immune system. Herbal antivirals have gained increasing attention for their potential to target respiratory viruses and offer complementary therapeutic options.

Mechanisms of Action

Herbs possess a diverse array of bioactive compounds, including flavonoids, alkaloids, terpenoids, and polyphenols, which can exhibit antiviral properties through various mechanisms. Some of the primary mechanisms by which herbal antivirals target respiratory viruses include:

Inhibition of viral entry and attachment: Certain herbs contain compounds that can bind to viral surface proteins or cellular receptors, preventing the virus from entering and infecting host cells.

Disruption of viral replication: Some herbal compounds can interfere with the replication cycle of viruses by inhibiting viral enzymes or disrupting the synthesis of viral proteins and nucleic acids.

Modulation of the immune system: Many herbs have immunomodulatory properties, enhancing the body's natural defences against viral infections by stimulating the production of cytokines, activating immune cells, and regulating inflammatory responses.

Antioxidant and anti-inflammatory effects: Herbal antioxidants can neutralise free radicals and reduce oxidative stress, while anti-inflammatory compounds can alleviate symptoms associated with respiratory viral infections.

Promising Herbal Antivirals for Respiratory Viruses

While numerous herbs have been studied for their antiviral potential, some particularly promising options for targeting respiratory viruses include:

Elderberry (Sambucus nigra):

Traditionally used for influenza and respiratory infections.
Contains flavonoids and anthocyanins with antiviral and immunomodulatory activities.
May inhibit viral entry and replication, as well as reduce symptom severity and duration.

Echinacea (Echinacea purpurea):

Long history of use for supporting immune function and treating respiratory infections.
Contains alkylamides, polysaccharides, and other compounds with antiviral and immunomodulatory effects.
May be effective against influenza and respiratory syncytial virus (RSV).

Astragalus (Astragalus membranaceus):

A popular adaptogenic herb in traditional Chinese medicine.
Contains polysaccharides, saponins, and flavonoids with immunomodulatory and antiviral properties.
May help alleviate symptoms and enhance immune responses against respiratory viruses.

Licorice (Glycyrrhiza glabra):

Commonly used in traditional medicine for respiratory conditions.
Contains glycyrrhizin and other compounds with antiviral, anti-inflammatory, and immunomodulatory effects.
May inhibit viral entry and replication, as well as alleviate respiratory symptoms.

Andrographis (Andrographis paniculata):

A popular herb in Ayurvedic and traditional Chinese medicine.
Contains andrographolides and other compounds with antiviral, anti-inflammatory, and immunomodulatory activities.
May be effective against influenza and other respiratory viruses.

Dosage and Administration

The appropriate dosage and administration of herbal antivirals for respiratory viral infections can vary depending on the specific herb, formulation, and individual patient factors. It is essential to consult reliable sources, such as reputable herbal monographs, clinical studies, or experienced herbalists, to determine the appropriate dosage range and administration techniques.

Common administration methods for herbal antivirals targeting respiratory viruses include:

Oral administration:

Teas, infusions, capsules, tablets, tinctures, and liquid extracts.
Dosages may range from a few grams of dried herb per day to standardised extracts with specific concentrations of active compounds.

Topical application:
Inhalation of herbal steams or use of herbal throat sprays for sore throats and respiratory discomfort.

Combination formulas:

Many traditional herbal formulations combine multiple herbs to leverage their synergistic effects and target various stages of viral infections.

It is important to note that while herbal antivirals are generally considered safe when used appropriately, they can still interact with medications and potentially cause adverse effects. Consulting with qualified healthcare professionals, such as herbalists, naturopathic doctors, or integrative medicine practitioners, is strongly recommended, especially for individuals with underlying medical conditions or those taking prescription medications.

Integrative Approach

While herbal antivirals offer promising complementary options for targeting respiratory viruses, they should not be viewed as a replacement for conventional medical care or antiviral medications prescribed by healthcare professionals. An integrative approach that combines herbal remedies with conventional treatments, when appropriate, may offer the most comprehensive and effective strategy for managing respiratory viral infections.

This integrative approach involves open communication between patients and healthcare providers, allowing for the safe and appropriate integration of herbal antivirals into treatment plans. Healthcare providers can provide guidance on potential herb-drug interactions, dosage adjustments, and monitoring for potential adverse effects or contraindications.

Additionally, lifestyle factors, such as proper hydration, rest, and nutritional support, can complement the use of herbal antivirals and support overall immune function during respiratory viral infections.

Research and Future Directions

While the field of herbal antivirals for respiratory viruses holds significant promise, further research is essential to expand our understanding and establish evidence-based guidelines. Clinical studies evaluating the efficacy, safety, and optimal dosing of herbal antivirals are needed, as well as investigations into their mechanisms of action and potential synergistic effects when combined with conventional antiviral medications.

Furthermore, the development of standardised and quality-controlled herbal products is crucial to ensure consistent and reliable results. Advances in analytical techniques, such as metabolomics and network pharmacology, can provide insights into the intricate interactions between herbal compounds and biological pathways, informing the development of more targeted and effective formulations.

Conclusion

Respiratory viral infections pose a significant burden on global health, and the search for effective and complementary therapeutic options remains an ongoing pursuit. Herbal antivirals offer a promising approach, leveraging the rich diversity of bioactive compounds found in plants to target respiratory viruses through various mechanisms, including inhibiting viral entry and replication, modulating the immune system, and reducing inflammation.

While preliminary research has highlighted the potential of several herbs, such as elderberry, echinacea, astragalus, licorice, and andrographis, further clinical studies are needed to establish their efficacy, safety, and appropriate dosing guidelines. An integrative approach that combines herbal remedies with conventional medical care, when appropriate, may offer the most comprehensive and effective strategy for managing respiratory viral infections.

Combatting Gastrointestinal Viruses: Herbal Solutions for Digestive Health

Gastrointestinal viral infections, such as those caused by norovirus, rotavirus, and enteric adenoviruses, can significantly impact digestive health and overall well-being. These viruses can lead to unpleasant symptoms like nausea, vomiting, diarrhoea, and abdominal discomfort, potentially causing dehydration and nutrient deficiencies. While conventional antiviral medications are available for some gastrointestinal viruses, many individuals seek natural alternatives, particularly herbal remedies, to alleviate symptoms and support their digestive system's recovery.

Herbal antivirals have gained increasing attention for their potential to combat gastrointestinal viruses and promote digestive health. These natural remedies offer a comprehensive approach by targeting various mechanisms involved in viral infections and associated symptoms.

Mechanisms of Action

Herbs possess a diverse array of bioactive compounds, including flavonoids, tannins, alkaloids, and terpenoids, which can exhibit antiviral and gastrointestinal-protective properties through various mechanisms:

Inhibition of viral entry and attachment: Certain herbs contain compounds that can bind to viral surface proteins or cellular receptors, preventing the virus from entering and infecting the intestinal cells.

Disruption of viral replication: Some herbal compounds can interfere with the replication cycle of gastrointestinal viruses by inhibiting viral enzymes or disrupting the synthesis of viral proteins and nucleic acids.

Modulation of the immune system: Many herbs have immunomodulatory properties, enhancing the body's natural defences against viral infections by stimulating the production of cytokines and activating immune cells in the gut-associated lymphoid tissue (GALT).

Anti-inflammatory and antioxidant effects: Herbal antioxidants can neutralise free radicals and reduce oxidative stress, while anti-inflammatory compounds can alleviate gastrointestinal inflammation and associated symptoms.

Antimicrobial and prebiotic effects: Certain herbs possess antimicrobial properties that can help maintain a healthy gut microbiome, while others act as prebiotics, supporting the growth of beneficial gut bacteria.

Promising Herbal Antivirals for Gastrointestinal Viruses

While numerous herbs have been studied for their antiviral potential, some particularly promising options for combatting gastrointestinal viruses and promoting digestive health include:

Ginger (Zingiber officinale):

Traditionally used for digestive issues and nausea relief.
Contains compounds like gingerol and shogaol with antiviral, anti-inflammatory, and antiemetic properties.
May inhibit viral entry and replication, as well as alleviate symptoms like nausea and vomiting.

Licorice (Glycyrrhiza glabra):

Commonly used in traditional medicine for digestive disorders.
Contains glycyrrhizin and other compounds with antiviral, anti-inflammatory, and immunomodulatory effects.
May inhibit viral entry and replication, as well as protect the gastrointestinal mucosa.

Cranberry (Vaccinium macrocarpon):

Well-known for its antimicrobial and antioxidant properties.
Contains proanthocyanidins and other compounds with antiviral and gastrointestinal-protective effects.
May inhibit viral attachment and replication, as well as support a healthy gut microbiome.

Turmeric (Curcuma longa):

A popular spice with a long history of use in traditional medicine.
Contains curcumin, a potent antioxidant and anti-inflammatory compound.
May alleviate gastrointestinal inflammation and support immune function during viral infections.

Marshmallow (Althaea officinalis):

Traditionally used for its soothing and protective effects on the digestive tract.

Contains mucilage and other compounds with anti-inflammatory and prebiotic properties.
May alleviate gastrointestinal discomfort and support a healthy gut microbiome.

Dosage and Administration

The appropriate dosage and administration of herbal antivirals for gastrointestinal viral infections can vary depending on the specific herb, formulation, and individual patient factors. It is essential to consult reliable sources, such as reputable herbal monographs, clinical studies, or experienced herbalists, to determine the appropriate dosage range and administration techniques.

Common administration methods for herbal antivirals targeting gastrointestinal viruses include:

Oral administration:

Teas, infusions, capsules, tablets, tinctures, and liquid extracts.
Dosages may range from a few grams of dried herb per day to standardised extracts with specific concentrations of active compounds.

Combination formulas:

Many traditional herbal formulations combine multiple herbs to leverage their synergistic effects and target various aspects of gastrointestinal health during viral infections.
It is important to note that while herbal antivirals are generally considered safe when used appropriately, they can still interact with medications and potentially cause adverse effects. Consulting with qualified healthcare professionals, such as herbalists, naturopathic doctors, or integrative medicine practitioners, is strongly recommended, especially for

individuals with underlying medical conditions or those taking prescription medications.

Integrative Approach and Supportive Measures

While herbal antivirals offer promising complementary options for combatting gastrointestinal viruses, they should be used in conjunction with supportive measures to address dehydration, electrolyte imbalances, and nutrient deficiencies that can occur during viral infections.

An integrative approach that combines herbal remedies with conventional treatments, when appropriate, and supportive measures may offer the most comprehensive and effective strategy for managing gastrointestinal viral infections. This approach involves open communication between patients and healthcare providers, allowing for the safe and appropriate integration of herbal antivirals into treatment plans.

Supportive measures may include:

Hydration: Consuming adequate fluids, such as water, electrolyte-balanced solutions, or herbal teas, to prevent dehydration.
Nutritional support: Consuming easily digestible, nutrient-dense foods and supplements to replenish essential nutrients and support recovery.
Probiotics: Introducing beneficial bacteria through probiotic supplements or fermented foods to support a healthy gut microbiome.
Rest and stress management: Allowing the body to rest and recover, while implementing stress-reduction techniques to support overall well-being.

Research and Future Directions

While the field of herbal antivirals for gastrointestinal viruses holds significant promise, further research is essential to expand our understanding and establish evidence-based guidelines. Clinical studies evaluating the efficacy, safety, and optimal dosing of herbal antivirals are needed, as well as investigations into their mechanisms of action and potential synergistic effects when combined with conventional antiviral medications or supportive therapies.

Furthermore, the development of standardised and quality-controlled herbal products is crucial to ensure consistent and reliable results. Advances in analytical techniques, such as metabolomics and network pharmacology, can provide insights into the intricate interactions between herbal compounds and biological pathways, informing the development of more targeted and effective formulations.

Conclusion

Gastrointestinal viral infections can have a significant impact on digestive health and overall well-being. Herbal antivirals offer a promising approach to combating these viruses and promoting digestive health, leveraging the rich diversity of bioactive compounds found in plants to target various mechanisms involved in viral infections and associated symptoms.

While preliminary research has highlighted the potential of several herbs, such as ginger, licorice, cranberry, turmeric, and marshmallow, further clinical studies are needed to establish their efficacy, safety, and appropriate dosing guidelines. An integrative approach that combines herbal remedies with supportive measures and conventional medical care, when appropriate, may offer the most comprehensive and effective strategy for managing gastrointestinal viral infections.

Herbs for Skin and Mucosal Viral Infections: Warts, Herpes, and More

Viral infections affecting the skin and mucosal surfaces can be challenging to treat and often recur, causing significant discomfort and distress. From the unsightly appearance of warts caused by human papillomavirus (HPV) to the painful outbreaks of herpes simplex virus (HSV), these viral infections can impact various aspects of an individual's life. While conventional antiviral medications are available, many individuals seek natural alternatives, particularly herbal remedies, to address these conditions.

Herbal antivirals have gained increasing attention for their potential to combat skin and mucosal viral infections, offering complementary therapeutic options. These natural remedies can target various mechanisms involved in viral infections and provide additional benefits, such as soothing inflammation and promoting healing.

Mechanisms of Action

Herbs possess a diverse array of bioactive compounds, including flavonoids, tannins, alkaloids, and terpenoids, which can exhibit antiviral and tissue-protective properties through various mechanisms:

Inhibition of viral entry and attachment: Certain herbs contain compounds that can bind to viral surface proteins or cellular receptors, preventing the virus from entering and infecting the skin or mucosal cells.

Disruption of viral replication: Some herbal compounds can interfere with the replication cycle of viruses by inhibiting viral enzymes or disrupting the synthesis of viral proteins and nucleic acids.

Modulation of the immune system: Many herbs have immunomodulatory properties, enhancing the body's natural defences against viral infections by stimulating the production of cytokines and activating immune cells.

Anti-inflammatory and antioxidant effects: Herbal antioxidants can neutralise free radicals and reduce oxidative stress, while anti-inflammatory compounds can alleviate inflammation and associated symptoms.

Tissue healing and regeneration: Certain herbs possess wound-healing and tissue-regenerative properties, which can aid in the recovery process and reduce scarring or tissue damage caused by viral infections.

Promising Herbal Antivirals for Skin and Mucosal Viral Infections

While numerous herbs have been studied for their antiviral potential, some particularly promising options for combatting skin and mucosal viral infections include:

Green Tea (Camellia sinensis):
Rich in polyphenolic compounds, such as epigallocatechin gallate (EGCG), with antiviral and anti-inflammatory properties.

May inhibit viral entry and replication, as well as alleviate inflammation and promote wound healing.
Potential applications for warts, herpes simplex virus (HSV), and other skin and mucosal viral infections.

Lemon Balm (Melissa officinalis):

Traditionally used for its antiviral and soothing properties.
Contains compounds like rosmarinic acid and terpenes with antiviral and anti-inflammatory effects.
May inhibit viral replication and alleviate symptoms associated with herpes simplex virus (HSV) infections.

Thyme (Thymus vulgaris):
A popular culinary herb with antimicrobial and antiviral properties.
Contains thymol, carvacrol, and other compounds with antiviral and anti-inflammatory effects.

May be effective against warts, herpes simplex virus (HSV), and other skin and mucosal viral infections.

Echinacea (Echinacea purpurea):
Well-known for its immunomodulatory and antiviral properties.
Contains alkylamides, polysaccharides, and other compounds with antiviral and wound-healing effects.
May enhance immune responses and promote tissue regeneration in viral skin and mucosal infections.

St. John's Wort (Hypericum perforatum):
A popular herb with antiviral and anti-inflammatory properties.
Contains hypericin, hyperforin, and other compounds with antiviral and wound-healing effects.
May inhibit viral replication and promote tissue healing in skin and mucosal viral infections.

Dosage and Administration

The appropriate dosage and administration of herbal antivirals for skin and mucosal viral infections can vary depending on the specific herb, formulation, and individual patient factors. It is essential to consult reliable sources, such as reputable herbal monographs, clinical studies, or experienced herbalists, to determine the appropriate dosage range and administration techniques.

Common administration methods for herbal antivirals targeting skin and mucosal viral infections include:

Topical application:

Ointments, creams, gels, or herbal extracts applied directly to the affected areas.
Specific herbs or combinations may be used for different viral infections.

Oral administration:

Teas, infusions, capsules, tablets, tinctures, and liquid extracts for systemic effects.
Dosages may range from a few grams of dried herb per day to standardised extracts with specific concentrations of active compounds.

Combination formulas:

Many traditional herbal formulations combine multiple herbs to leverage their synergistic effects and target various aspects of skin and mucosal viral infections.
It is important to note that while herbal antivirals are generally considered safe when used appropriately, they can still interact with medications and potentially cause adverse effects. Consulting with qualified healthcare professionals, such as herbalists, naturopathic doctors, or integrative medicine practitioners, is strongly recommended, especially for individuals with underlying medical

conditions or those taking prescription medications.

Integrative Approach and Supportive Measures

While herbal antivirals offer promising complementary options for combatting skin and mucosal viral infections, they should be used in conjunction with supportive measures to promote healing, alleviate discomfort, and prevent complications.

An integrative approach that combines herbal remedies with conventional treatments, when appropriate, and supportive measures may offer the most comprehensive and effective strategy for managing skin and mucosal viral infections. This approach involves open communication between patients and healthcare providers, allowing for the safe and appropriate integration of herbal antivirals into treatment plans.

Supportive measures may include:

Proper hygiene and wound care: Keeping affected areas clean and protected to prevent secondary infections and promote healing.

Stress management: Implementing stress-reduction techniques, as stress can exacerbate viral outbreaks and impair healing.

Nutritional support: Consuming a balanced diet rich in essential nutrients to support immune function and tissue regeneration.

Pain management: Using appropriate pain relief measures, such as over-the-counter or prescribed medications, to alleviate discomfort associated with viral infections.

Research and Future Directions

While the field of herbal antivirals for skin and mucosal viral infections holds significant promise, further research is essential to expand our understanding and establish evidence-based guidelines. Clinical studies evaluating the efficacy, safety, and optimal dosing of herbal antivirals are needed, as well as investigations into their mechanisms of action and potential synergistic effects when combined with conventional antiviral medications or supportive therapies.

Furthermore, the development of standardised and quality-controlled herbal products is crucial to ensure consistent and reliable results. Advances in analytical techniques, such as metabolomics and network pharmacology, can provide insights into the intricate interactions between herbal compounds and biological pathways, informing the development of more targeted and effective formulations.

Conclusion

Skin and mucosal viral infections like warts, herpes, and others can significantly impact an individual's quality of life and overall well-being. Herbal antivirals offer a promising approach to combating these viruses, leveraging the rich diversity of bioactive compounds found in plants to target various mechanisms involved in viral infections and associated symptoms.

While preliminary research has highlighted the potential of several herbs, such as green tea, lemon balm, thyme, echinacea, and St. John's wort, further clinical studies are needed to establish their efficacy, safety, and appropriate dosing guidelines. An integrative approach that combines herbal remedies with supportive measures and conventional medical care, when appropriate, may offer the most comprehensive and effective strategy for managing skin and mucosal viral infections.

Chapter 5: Enhancing Immunity and Long-Term Wellness

Holistic Approaches to Immune Support: Herbs, Nutrition, and Lifestyle

Maintaining a robust and well-functioning immune system is crucial for overall health and well-being, especially in the face of viral infections. While conventional antiviral medications play a vital role in the management of many viral diseases, a growing body of evidence suggests that a holistic approach, combining herbal remedies, proper nutrition, and a healthy lifestyle, can significantly enhance immune function and support the body's natural defences.

Herbal Antivirals and Immune Support

Herbs have been used for centuries in traditional medicine systems around the world for their immune-boosting properties. Many herbs contain a diverse array of bioactive compounds, such as polyphenols, alkaloids, and terpenoids, which can modulate the immune system through various mechanisms:

Immunomodulation: Certain herbs possess compounds that can stimulate the production of cytokines, activate immune cells like macrophages and natural killer cells, and enhance the body's overall immune response to viral infections.

Anti-inflammatory effects: Inflammation can compromise immune function, and many herbs contain potent anti-inflammatory compounds that can help regulate immune responses and reduce tissue damage associated with viral infections.

Antioxidant properties: Oxidative stress can weaken the immune system, and herbs rich in antioxidants can help neutralise free radicals and protect immune cells from oxidative damage.

Some promising herbs for immune support and their potential mechanisms include:

Astragalus (Astragalus membranaceus): Enhances immune cell function and stimulates cytokine production.

Echinacea (Echinacea purpurea): Modulates immune responses, stimulates macrophage activity, and possesses antiviral properties.

Elderberry (Sambucus nigra): Rich in antioxidants and immunomodulatory compounds, with potential antiviral effects.

Turmeric (Curcuma longa): Provides potent anti-inflammatory and antioxidant support due to its curcumin content.

Nutritional Support for Immune Function

A balanced and nutrient-dense diet plays a crucial role in supporting immune function and enhancing the body's defences against viral infections. Key nutrients and their roles in immune support include:

Vitamins:

Vitamin C: A powerful antioxidant that supports immune cell function and enhances antiviral responses.
Vitamin D: Regulates immune cell activity and has been linked to reduced risk of respiratory infections.
Vitamin E: An antioxidant that protects immune cells from oxidative stress.

Minerals:

Zinc: Essential for immune cell development and function, as well as antiviral and anti-inflammatory activities.

Selenium: Supports immune cell proliferation and function, with antioxidant properties.

Omega-3 fatty acids: Found in fatty fish, nuts, and seeds, omega-3s possess anti-inflammatory properties and support immune cell function.

Probiotics and prebiotics: A healthy gut microbiome is crucial for immune function, and probiotic and prebiotic foods can support a balanced gut microbiota.

Lifestyle Factors and Immune Health

In addition to herbs and nutrition, various lifestyle factors play a significant role in maintaining a robust immune system and supporting the body's defences against viral infections:

Stress management: Chronic stress can suppress immune function, making it essential to incorporate stress-reducing practices like meditation, yoga, or mindfulness exercises into daily routines.

Sleep and rest: Adequate sleep and rest are vital for immune cell regeneration and function. Aim for 7-9 hours of quality sleep per night.

Exercise and physical activity: Regular moderate exercise can enhance immune cell circulation and function, while excessive or intense exercise can be immunosuppressive.

Smoking cessation and alcohol moderation: Smoking and excessive alcohol consumption can impair immune function and increase the risk of respiratory infections.

Environmental factors: Exposure to toxins, pollutants, and allergens can contribute to inflammation and compromise immune responses.

Integrative and Holistic Approach

While herbal remedies, proper nutrition, and a healthy lifestyle can provide significant immune support, it is essential to integrate these holistic approaches with conventional medical care when appropriate. Open communication between patients and healthcare providers is crucial to ensure the safe and appropriate integration of herbal antivirals, dietary supplements, and lifestyle modifications into treatment plans.

Healthcare professionals, such as herbalists, naturopathic doctors, and integrative medicine practitioners, can provide guidance on:

Selecting appropriate herbal formulations and dosages based on individual needs and potential interactions with medications.

Developing personalised dietary plans and supplement recommendations to address nutrient deficiencies and support immune function.

Implementing lifestyle changes and stress management techniques tailored to individual circumstances.

Monitoring progress and adjusting strategies as needed for optimal immune support and viral management.

Research and Future Directions

While the field of herbal antivirals and holistic immune support holds significant promise, further research is essential to expand our understanding and establish evidence-based guidelines. Clinical studies evaluating the efficacy, safety, and optimal dosing of herbal antivirals and nutrient-based interventions are needed, as well as investigations into their mechanisms of action and potential synergistic effects with conventional antiviral medications.

Furthermore, the development of standardised and quality-controlled herbal and dietary supplement products is crucial to ensure consistent and reliable results. Advances in analytical techniques, such as metabolomics and network pharmacology, can provide insights into the intricate interactions between natural compounds, biological pathways, and immune function, informing the development of more targeted and effective formulations.

Conclusion

Maintaining a robust immune system is crucial in the fight against viral infections, and a holistic approach that combines herbal antivirals, proper nutrition, and a healthy lifestyle can provide comprehensive support. By leveraging the synergistic effects of these complementary strategies, individuals can enhance their body's natural defences, reduce the risk of viral infections, and support overall health and well-being.

As we continue to explore the potential of herbal antivirals and holistic immune support, it is essential to promote responsible use, quality control, and open communication between patients and healthcare providers. By embracing the wisdom of traditional medicine and integrating it with modern scientific understanding, we can unlock the full potential of natural compounds and lifestyle interventions in our efforts to combat viral infections and promote optimal immune function.

Adaptogens: Herbs for Stress Resilience and Immune Balance

In the fast-paced and demanding world we live in, stress has become an inevitable part of our lives. Chronic stress can have profound effects on our overall well-being, including suppressing immune function and increasing susceptibility to viral infections. To combat the negative impacts of stress, many individuals are turning to adaptogens – a unique class of herbs that have been used for centuries in traditional medicine systems for their ability to help the body adapt to and resist various forms of stress.

What are Adaptogens?

Adaptogens are non-toxic plants that are known to help the body cope with physical, mental, and environmental stressors. These herbs are believed to work by modulating the body's stress response system, particularly the hypothalamic-pituitary-adrenal (HPA) axis, which plays a crucial role in regulating immune function, energy levels, and overall homeostasis.

Mechanisms of Action

Adaptogens exhibit a wide range of beneficial effects on the body, including:

Immunomodulation: Many adaptogens possess immunomodulatory properties, helping to balance and optimise immune function. They can stimulate the production of immune cells and cytokines, enhancing the body's defences against viral infections and other pathogens.

Anti-inflammatory effects: Chronic stress and inflammation can suppress immune function and increase susceptibility to viral infections. Adaptogens contain compounds with potent anti-inflammatory properties, helping to reduce oxidative stress and regulate inflammatory responses.

Neuroprotective and anxiolytic effects: Adaptogens have been shown to have neuroprotective effects, helping to mitigate the negative impacts of stress on the brain and central nervous system. Some adaptogens also exhibit anxiolytic (anti-anxiety) properties, promoting a sense of calm and reducing stress-induced anxiety.

Metabolic regulation: Adaptogens can help regulate metabolic processes, supporting energy production, and promoting healthy glucose and lipid metabolism, which can be disrupted by chronic stress.

Promising Adaptogenic Herbs

While there are many herbs with adaptogenic properties, some of the most well-studied and promising options include:

Ashwagandha (Withania somnifera): A renowned adaptogen in Ayurvedic medicine, known for its immune-boosting and anti-stress effects.

May enhance immune cell function, modulate inflammatory responses, and promote a balanced stress response.

Rhodiola (Rhodiola rosea):

A popular adaptogen in traditional Russian and Scandinavian medicine, known for its ability to improve physical and mental performance under stress.
May support immune function, reduce inflammation, and enhance cognitive function and mood.

Eleuthero (Eleutherococcus senticosus):
Also known as Siberian ginseng, this adaptogen has been used in traditional Chinese medicine for its tonifying properties.
May enhance immune responses, reduce fatigue, and improve physical and mental performance under stress.

Reishi (Ganoderma lucidum):

A revered medicinal mushroom in traditional Chinese medicine, with adaptogenic and immune-modulating properties.
May support immune function, reduce inflammation, and promote a balanced stress response.

Holy Basil (Ocimum tenuiflorum):

A sacred herb in Ayurvedic medicine, known for its ability to promote resilience and balance during times of stress.
May enhance immune function, reduce inflammation, and promote a sense of calm and well-being.

Integrating Adaptogens into a Holistic Approach

While adaptogens offer promising benefits for stress resilience and immune balance, it is important to integrate them into a holistic approach that includes other lifestyle modifications and supportive measures. This comprehensive strategy can help maximise the effectiveness of adaptogens and promote overall well-being.

Stress management techniques: Incorporating practices such as meditation, yoga, deep breathing exercises, and mindfulness can help reduce stress levels and promote relaxation.

Balanced nutrition: A nutrient-dense diet rich in whole foods, antioxidants, and anti-inflammatory compounds can support immune function and help mitigate the effects of stress on the body.

Regular exercise: Engaging in moderate physical activity can help reduce stress, boost mood, and promote overall health and well-being.

Adequate sleep and rest: Getting sufficient sleep and allowing the body to rest and recover is essential for stress resilience and immune balance.

Professional guidance: Consulting with qualified healthcare professionals, such as herbalists, naturopathic doctors, or integrative medicine practitioners, can help ensure the safe and appropriate use of adaptogens and other complementary therapies.

Research and Future Directions

While the field of adaptogenic herbs and their applications in stress resilience and immune balance holds significant promise, further research is essential to expand our understanding and establish evidence-based guidelines. Clinical studies evaluating the efficacy, safety, and optimal dosing of adaptogens are needed, as well as investigations into their mechanisms of action and potential synergistic effects with other natural compounds or conventional therapies.

Furthermore, the development of standardised and quality-controlled adaptogenic products is crucial to ensure consistent and reliable results. Advances in analytical techniques, such as metabolomics and network pharmacology, can provide insights into the intricate interactions between adaptogenic compounds, biological pathways, and the stress response system, informing the development of more targeted and effective formulations.

Conclusion

In the face of modern-day stressors and the challenges posed by viral infections, adaptogens offer a promising natural approach to enhance stress resilience and immune balance. By modulating the body's stress response system, regulating immune function, and exhibiting anti-inflammatory and neuroprotective effects, these remarkable herbs can help the body adapt and cope with various forms of stress.

As we continue to explore the potential of adaptogens, it is essential to promote responsible use, quality control, and open communication between patients and healthcare providers. By integrating these powerful herbs into a holistic approach that includes lifestyle modifications and supportive measures, we can unlock their full potential in promoting overall well-being and resilience in the face of stress and viral challenges.

Longevity and Vitality: Herbs for Overall Well-Being

In the pursuit of a long and healthy life, individuals are increasingly seeking natural and holistic approaches to promote overall well-being. While modern medicine has made remarkable strides in treating diseases and extending lifespan, many are turning to the ancient wisdom of herbal remedies to support longevity and vitality. Herbs have been revered for centuries in various traditional medicine systems for their ability to fortify the body, enhance resilience, and promote a balanced state of being.

The Concept of Longevity and Vitality

Longevity refers to the duration of life, while vitality encompasses the state of being full of life, energy, and vigour. Together, these concepts represent the ultimate goal of achieving a long and vibrant life, free from debilitating diseases and age-related declines. Herbs have the potential to contribute to this goal by targeting various mechanisms that influence longevity and vitality:

Antioxidant and anti-inflammatory properties: Many herbs are rich in antioxidants and possess anti-inflammatory compounds that can help protect cells and tissues from oxidative stress and chronic inflammation, both of which are implicated in ageing and various age-related diseases.

Immunomodulatory effects: Herbs can help modulate and optimise immune function, supporting the body's natural defences against pathogens, infections, and age-related immune dysregulation.

Adaptogenic and stress-resilience properties: Certain herbs, known as adaptogens, can help the body adapt to and resist various forms of stress, including physical, mental, and environmental stressors, which can contribute to accelerated ageing and declining vitality.

Neuroprotective and cognitive-enhancing effects: Some herbs have been shown to possess neuroprotective properties, helping to preserve cognitive function and potentially delaying or preventing age-related neurodegenerative diseases.

Metabolic regulation and hormonal balance: Herbs can help regulate metabolic processes, support healthy glucose and lipid metabolism, and promote hormonal balance, all of which are crucial for overall health and vitality as we age.

Promising Herbs for Longevity and Vitality

While numerous herbs have been explored for their potential benefits in promoting longevity and vitality, some particularly promising options include:

Ginseng (Panax ginseng):

A revered adaptogenic herb in traditional Chinese medicine, known for its tonifying and rejuvenating properties.

May enhance energy levels, support cognitive function, and promote overall well-being.

Turmeric (Curcuma longa):

A vibrant spice with a long history of use in Ayurvedic medicine, renowned for its potent antioxidant and anti-inflammatory properties.
May help protect against various age-related diseases and support healthy ageing.

Ashwagandha (Withania somnifera):
An adaptogenic herb in Ayurveda, valued for its ability to promote resilience and balance in the face of stress.
May support immune function, cognitive health, and overall vitality.

Ginkgo (Ginkgo biloba):
An ancient tree species with a long history of use in traditional Chinese medicine for its neuroprotective and cognitive-enhancing properties.

May improve cerebral blood flow, support brain function, and potentially delay age-related cognitive decline.

Rhodiola (Rhodiola rosea):
A renowned adaptogenic herb in traditional Russian and Scandinavian medicine, known for its ability to enhance physical and mental performance under stress.
May support energy levels, cognitive function, and overall resilience.

Integrating Herbs into a Holistic Lifestyle

While herbs offer promising benefits for promoting longevity and vitality, it is important to integrate them into a holistic lifestyle approach that includes other supportive measures. This comprehensive strategy can help maximise the effectiveness of herbs and promote overall well-being:

Balanced nutrition: A nutrient-dense diet rich in whole foods, antioxidants, and anti-inflammatory compounds can complement the benefits of herbs and support overall health and longevity.

Regular exercise: Engaging in moderate physical activity can help maintain cardiovascular health, promote muscle and bone strength, and support cognitive function, all of which contribute to longevity and vitality.

Stress management: Incorporating practices such as meditation, yoga, deep breathing exercises, and mindfulness can help reduce stress levels and promote relaxation, supporting overall resilience and well-being.

Adequate sleep and rest: Getting sufficient sleep and allowing the body to rest and recover is essential for maintaining energy levels, cognitive function, and overall vitality.

Social connections and purpose: Maintaining strong social connections and cultivating a sense of purpose can contribute to mental and emotional well-being, which are important factors in overall longevity and vitality.

Professional guidance: Consulting with qualified healthcare professionals, such as herbalists, naturopathic doctors, or integrative medicine practitioners, can help ensure the safe and appropriate use of herbs and other complementary therapies.

Research and Future Directions

While the field of herbal medicine and its applications in promoting longevity and vitality hold significant promise, further research is essential to expand our understanding and establish evidence-based guidelines. Clinical studies evaluating the efficacy, safety, and optimal dosing of longevity-promoting herbs are needed, as well as investigations into their mechanisms of action and potential synergistic effects with other natural compounds or conventional therapies.

Furthermore, the development of standardised and quality-controlled herbal products is crucial to ensure consistent and reliable results. Advances in analytical techniques, such as metabolomics and network pharmacology, can provide insights into the intricate interactions between herbal compounds, biological pathways, and the ageing process, informing the development of more targeted and effective formulations.

Conclusion

In the pursuit of a long and vibrant life, herbs offer a promising natural approach to promote longevity and vitality. By harnessing the power of antioxidants, anti-inflammatory compounds, immunomodulatory effects, adaptogenic properties, and neuroprotective mechanisms, these remarkable plants can support overall well-being and potentially delay or prevent age-related declines.

Embracing the wisdom of traditional medicine systems and integrating it with modern scientific understanding, we can pave the way for a future where longevity and vitality are not just aspirations but attainable realities for all.

Chapter 6: Special Considerations and Safety Guidelines

Herbal Medicine for Pregnancy and Breastfeeding

The journey of pregnancy and breastfeeding is a remarkable and transformative experience for many women. During this time, maintaining optimal health and well-being is of paramount importance, not only for the mother but also for the developing foetus or nursing infant. While conventional medicine offers valuable support, many expectant and breastfeeding mothers seek complementary approaches, including herbal remedies, to address various concerns and promote overall wellness.

Herbal medicines have been used for centuries in traditional healing systems to support women's health during pregnancy and lactation. However, it is crucial to navigate the use of herbal remedies with caution and guidance, as some herbs may pose potential risks or have unintended consequences during these delicate life stages.

Safety Considerations

The safety of herbal medicines during pregnancy and breastfeeding is a primary concern. The developing foetus and nursing infant are particularly vulnerable to the effects of any substances ingested by the mother. Several factors must be carefully evaluated:

Teratogenic potential: Some herbs may have teratogenic effects, meaning they can cause birth defects or developmental abnormalities in the foetus if consumed during certain stages of pregnancy.

Uterine stimulant effects: Certain herbs may possess uterine stimulant properties, which could potentially increase the risk of preterm labour or miscarriage if consumed during pregnancy.

Transfer to breast milk: Herbs and their active compounds can potentially transfer into breast milk, potentially affecting the nursing infant's health and development.

Herb-drug interactions: Herbal remedies may interact with prescription medications, potentially altering their efficacy or increasing the risk of adverse effects.

It is crucial to consult with qualified healthcare professionals, such as herbalists, midwives, or integrative medicine practitioners, to evaluate the safety of specific herbs for each individual case, considering factors such as the stage of pregnancy, underlying health conditions, and concomitant medications.

Potential Applications and Promising Herbs

While caution is warranted, there are instances where herbal remedies may offer valuable support during pregnancy and breastfeeding when used appropriately and under professional guidance. Some potential applications and promising herbs include:

Morning sickness and nausea: Ginger (Zingiber officinale) has been traditionally used to alleviate morning sickness and nausea during pregnancy.
Red raspberry leaf (Rubus idaeus) may help reduce nausea and vomiting in early pregnancy.
Nutritional support: Herbs like nettle (Urtica dioica) and red raspberry leaf can provide essential nutrients and support during pregnancy and lactation.
Fenugreek (Trigonella foenum-graecum) may help increase breast milk production in nursing mothers.

Labour preparation and support: Herbs like red raspberry leaf and evening primrose oil (Oenothera biennis) have been traditionally used to prepare the uterus for labour, although their efficacy is still being researched.

Postpartum recovery: Herbs like ashwagandha (Withania somnifera) and rhodiola (Rhodiola rosea) may help support postpartum recovery and address issues like fatigue and stress.

It is important to note that while some herbs may offer potential benefits, others should be strictly avoided during pregnancy and breastfeeding due to their potential risks. Examples of herbs that are generally contraindicated include black cohosh, blue cohosh, dong quai, and pennyroyal.

Integrative Approach and Professional Guidance

Herbal medicine should be approached as a complementary therapy during pregnancy and breastfeeding, not a replacement for conventional medical care. An integrative approach that combines the expertise of healthcare professionals, such as obstetricians, midwives, herbalists, and integrative medicine practitioners, is crucial to ensure the safe and appropriate use of herbal remedies.

Healthcare professionals can provide guidance on:

Evaluating the safety and efficacy of specific herbs based on the individual's medical history, stage of pregnancy or lactation, and potential herb-drug interactions.

Recommending appropriate dosages and administration techniques for safe and effective use of herbal remedies.

Monitoring the mother's and infant's health and adjusting herbal protocols as needed throughout the pregnancy and breastfeeding journey.

Addressing potential concerns or adverse effects related to herbal use and providing timely intervention if necessary.

Additionally, it is essential to prioritise the use of high-quality, standardised herbal products from reputable sources to ensure consistent and reliable results.

Research and Future Directions

While the field of herbal medicine for pregnancy and breastfeeding holds promise, further research is essential to establish evidence-based guidelines and expand our understanding of the safety and efficacy of specific herbs during these critical life stages.

Clinical studies evaluating the effects of herbal remedies on maternal and foetal/infant health are needed, as well as investigations into potential herb-drug interactions and optimal dosing regimens.

Additionally, the development of standardised and quality-controlled herbal products specifically formulated for use during pregnancy and breastfeeding is crucial to ensure consistent and reliable results.

Advances in analytical techniques, such as metabolomics and pharmacokinetic studies, can provide insights into the transfer of herbal compounds from mother to foetus or breast milk, informing the development of safer and more targeted herbal formulations.

Conclusion

Herbal medicine can offer valuable complementary support during the transformative journey of pregnancy and breastfeeding. However, navigating the safety and efficacy of herbal remedies during these delicate life stages requires careful consideration and professional guidance.

By prioritising safety, consulting with qualified healthcare professionals, and following an integrative approach, expectant and breastfeeding mothers can potentially benefit from the therapeutic properties of selected herbs while minimising potential risks to themselves and their developing or nursing infants.

Paediatric Herbalism: Gentle Remedies for Children

Children's health and well-being are of paramount importance, and parents often seek natural and gentle alternatives to conventional medications, particularly for minor ailments and preventative care. Herbal remedies have been used for centuries in traditional medicine systems to support children's health, offering a holistic approach that many families find appealing. However, when it comes to paediatric herbalism, special considerations must be taken into account to ensure the safety and efficacy of these natural remedies.

Safety Considerations in Pediatric Herbalism

Children's bodies are still developing, and their metabolic processes and organ systems differ from those of adults. As such, the use of herbal remedies in paediatric populations requires extra caution and careful evaluation of potential risks and benefits:

Dosage adjustments: Children's smaller body size and weight necessitate appropriate dosage adjustments to prevent overdosing or adverse effects.

Developmental stage: The safety and suitability of certain herbs may vary depending on the child's age and developmental stage, as their physiological processes and potential sensitivities change over time.

Herb-drug interactions: If a child is taking prescribed medications, it is essential to consider potential herb-drug interactions that could alter the effectiveness or increase the risk of side effects.

Quality and purity: Children are particularly vulnerable to contaminants or adulterants in herbal products, emphasising the importance of using high-quality, standardised, and properly sourced herbal remedies.

It is crucial to consult with qualified healthcare professionals, such as herbalists, naturopathic doctors, or integrative paediatricians, to ensure the safe and appropriate use of herbal remedies for children.

Promising Herbal Remedies for Children

While caution is warranted, many herbs have been traditionally used to support children's health and well-being when administered appropriately. Some promising herbal remedies for common childhood conditions include:

Respiratory Support:

Elderberry (Sambucus nigra): Rich in antioxidants and immunomodulatory compounds, it may help alleviate symptoms of colds and flu.
Thyme (Thymus vulgaris): Possesses antimicrobial and expectorant properties,

potentially beneficial for respiratory infections and coughs.

Digestive Health:

Fennel (Foeniculum vulgare): May help relieve digestive discomfort, gas, and colic in infants and young children.
Chamomile (Matricaria chamomilla): Known for its soothing and anti-inflammatory properties, it can be helpful for digestive issues and teething discomfort.

Immune Support:

Echinacea (Echinacea purpurea): May help stimulate the immune system and reduce the duration and severity of respiratory infections.
Astragalus (Astragalus membranaceus): An adaptogenic herb with immunomodulatory properties that can support overall immune function.

Relaxation and Sleep:

Chamomile (Matricaria chamomilla): Its mild sedative effects can promote relaxation and improve sleep quality in children.

Lemon balm (Melissa officinalis): May help reduce anxiety and promote calmness in children.

Appropriate Administration and Preparation

The administration and preparation of herbal remedies for children require special considerations to ensure palatability, accurate dosing, and safe consumption:

Paediatric dosage forms: Herbal teas, glycerites (alcohol-free herbal extracts), and syrups are commonly used for children, as they are generally more palatable and easier to administer than capsules or tablets.

Taste and flavour: Children may be more sensitive to bitter or unpleasant tastes, so herbs with milder flavours or those combined with natural sweeteners or fruit juices may be preferable.

Safety precautions: Proper sterilisation of equipment and preparation surfaces is essential, especially for infants and young children with developing immune systems.

Parental guidance: Clear instructions and supervision from parents or caregivers are crucial to ensure correct administration and avoid potential misuse or accidental ingestion.

Integrative Approach and Professional Guidance

Herbal remedies should be used as complementary therapies, not as replacements for conventional medical care, especially in cases of serious or acute illnesses. An integrative approach that combines the expertise of healthcare professionals, such as paediatricians, herbalists, and integrative medicine practitioners, is essential for ensuring the safe and appropriate use of herbal remedies for children.

Healthcare professionals can provide guidance on:

Evaluating the suitability and safety of specific herbs based on the child's age, health condition, and potential herb-drug interactions.

Recommending appropriate dosages and administration techniques tailored to the child's needs and preferences.

Monitoring the child's health and adjusting herbal protocols as needed throughout their growth and development.

Addressing potential concerns or adverse effects related to herbal use and providing timely intervention if necessary.

Additionally, it is crucial to prioritise the use of high-quality, standardised herbal products from reputable sources to ensure consistent and reliable results.

Research and Future Directions

While the field of paediatric herbalism holds promise, further research is essential to establish evidence-based guidelines and expand our understanding of the safety and efficacy of specific herbs for children at different developmental stages.

Clinical studies evaluating the effects of herbal remedies on children's health and well-being are needed, as well as investigations into potential herb-drug interactions and optimal dosing regimens. Additionally, the development of standardised and quality-controlled herbal products specifically formulated for paediatric use is crucial to ensure consistent and reliable results.

Advances in analytical techniques and pharmacokinetic studies can provide insights into the absorption, distribution, metabolism, and excretion of herbal compounds in children, informing the development of safer and more targeted herbal formulations.

Conclusion

Paediatric herbalism offers a gentle and holistic approach to supporting children's health and well-being. By carefully considering safety factors, selecting appropriate herbal remedies, and ensuring proper administration techniques, parents and healthcare professionals can potentially benefit from the therapeutic properties of selected herbs while minimising potential risks.

An integrative approach that combines the wisdom of traditional healing systems with modern scientific understanding and professional guidance is essential for navigating the safe and effective use of herbal remedies for children. By prioritising quality control, conducting further research, and fostering open communication between parents and healthcare providers, we can pave the way for safer and more effective herbal solutions that support the overall well-being of our youngest generation.

Contraindications and Precautions: Using Herbal Antivirals Wisely

Herbal antivirals have gained increasing popularity as complementary or alternative options for managing viral infections and supporting overall health. While many herbs offer promising therapeutic benefits, it is crucial to recognize that they are not without potential risks and contraindications. Like any other therapeutic intervention, the use of herbal antivirals requires careful consideration, caution, and professional guidance to ensure their safe and effective use.

Contraindications and Potential Risks

Contraindications refer to specific situations or conditions where the use of a particular herb or herbal formulation is inadvisable or should be avoided altogether. Understanding these contraindications is essential to mitigate potential risks and prevent adverse effects.

Some common contraindications and potential risks associated with herbal antivirals include:

Herb-Drug Interactions: Many herbs and their active compounds can interact with prescription medications, over-the-counter drugs, and even other herbal supplements. These interactions can potentially alter the efficacy of the drugs, increase the risk of side effects, or cause adverse reactions. It is crucial to disclose all medications and supplements to healthcare providers to evaluate potential interactions.

Pregnancy and Lactation: During pregnancy and breastfeeding, the use of certain herbs should be approached with extreme caution or avoided altogether. Some herbal compounds can cross the placental barrier or be transferred through breast milk, potentially affecting the developing foetus or nursing infant. Consultation with qualified healthcare professionals is essential to evaluate the safety of specific herbs during these critical life stages.

Chronic Medical Conditions: Individuals with pre-existing medical conditions, such as liver or kidney disease, diabetes, or autoimmune disorders, may have altered metabolism or sensitivity to certain herbal compounds. These conditions may require dose adjustments or avoidance of specific herbs to prevent potential complications or exacerbation of the underlying condition.

Allergic Reactions: Like any substance, certain herbs can trigger allergic reactions in some individuals. It is important to be aware of potential allergies or sensitivities and to exercise caution when introducing new herbal remedies, especially those from the same plant family as known allergens.

Surgical Precautions: Some herbs may interact with anaesthetics or affect bleeding and clotting mechanisms, potentially increasing the risk of complications during and after surgical procedures. It is generally recommended to discontinue the use of herbal antivirals prior to surgery and consult with healthcare providers regarding the appropriate timing for resumption.

Precautions and Safe Use

In addition to understanding contraindications, adhering to certain precautions and guidelines can help ensure the safe and effective use of herbal antivirals:

Quality and Standardization: Choosing high-quality, standardised herbal products from reputable sources is crucial to ensure consistent potency, purity, and safety. Herbal products can vary significantly in their composition and concentration of active compounds, which can impact their efficacy and potential for adverse effects.

Proper Dosing: Adhering to appropriate dosage guidelines is essential to avoid potential toxicity or adverse effects. Overdosing on certain herbs can lead to unintended consequences, such as liver or kidney damage, or interactions with medications. Consulting with qualified healthcare professionals or referring to reliable sources for dosing information is recommended.

Duration of Use: Some herbal antivirals may be intended for short-term or acute use, while others may be suitable for longer-term or chronic use. Following recommended guidelines for duration of use can help prevent potential adverse effects associated with prolonged exposure to certain herbal compounds.

Monitoring and Reporting: When using herbal antivirals, it is important to monitor for any potential adverse effects or unexpected reactions. Keeping healthcare providers informed about the use of herbal remedies and reporting any concerns or adverse events is crucial for ensuring appropriate monitoring and adjustments to the treatment plan.

Professional Guidance: Consulting with qualified healthcare professionals, such as herbalists, naturopathic doctors, or integrative medicine practitioners, is strongly recommended when considering the use of herbal antivirals. These professionals can provide personalised guidance, evaluate potential contraindications and interactions, and ensure the safe and appropriate use of herbal remedies based on individual circumstances.

Integrative Approach and Patient Education

While herbal antivirals offer promising complementary options for managing viral infections, it is essential to approach their use with caution and as part of an integrative healthcare approach. Open communication between patients and healthcare providers is crucial to ensure the safe and appropriate integration of herbal antivirals into treatment plans.

Patient education plays a vital role in promoting the responsible use of herbal antivirals. Healthcare providers should provide clear information about potential contraindications, precautions, and proper usage guidelines. Encouraging patients to disclose all medications, supplements, and underlying medical conditions can help identify potential risks and facilitate informed decision-making.

Additionally, emphasising the importance of quality control, standardisation, and sourcing herbal products from reputable sources can help mitigate potential risks and ensure consistent and reliable results.

Research and Future Directions

While the field of herbal antivirals continues to evolve, further research is essential to expand our understanding of potential contraindications, herb-drug interactions, and safety profiles of specific herbs and herbal formulations. Clinical studies evaluating the efficacy, safety, and optimal dosing of herbal antivirals in various populations are needed, as well as investigations into potential adverse effects and long-term consequences of their use. Furthermore, the development of standardised and quality-controlled herbal products is crucial to ensure consistent and reliable results. Advances in analytical techniques, such as metabolomics and network pharmacology, can provide insights into the interactions between herbal compounds and biological pathways, informing the development of safer and more targeted herbal formulations.

Conclusion

Herbal antivirals offer promising therapeutic options for managing viral infections and supporting overall health, but their use must be approached with wisdom, caution, and professional guidance. Understanding potential contraindications, adhering to precautions, and maintaining open communication with healthcare providers are essential steps in ensuring the safe and effective use of these natural remedies.

By embracing an integrative approach that combines the wisdom of traditional medicine with modern scientific understanding, we can unlock the full potential of herbal antivirals while prioritising patient safety and responsible use. Through ongoing research, quality control, and patient education, we can pave the way for the responsible integration of herbal antivirals into healthcare practices, offering complementary and holistic solutions for promoting overall well-being.

Chapter 7: Herbal Antiviral Recipes: From Nature to Wellness

Welcome to a treasury of herbal wisdom passed down through generations, drawn from the archives of my beloved grandmother's herbal apothecary. In these pages, you will discover an array of potent herbal antiviral recipes, carefully crafted to harness the healing power of nature and bolster your body's defences against viral infections.

Throughout history, communities around the world have relied on the medicinal properties of plants to combat illness and promote well-being. My grandmother, a revered herbalist in her own right, dedicated her life to studying the therapeutic properties of herbs and sharing her knowledge with those in need. From soothing balms to invigorating teas, her herbal remedies have brought relief and comfort to countless individuals facing various health challenges.

In the face of today's global health concerns, the need for natural antiviral solutions has never been more urgent. As we navigate through uncertain times, it is essential to arm ourselves with the tools and knowledge necessary to support our immune systems and protect our health. The herbal antiviral recipes presented here offer a holistic approach to wellness, addressing not only the physical symptoms of viral infections but also nurturing the mind and spirit.

Derived from centuries of traditional wisdom and informed by modern scientific research, these recipes blend time-honoured herbal remedies with contemporary understanding to create powerful formulations for viral defence. Each recipe is carefully curated to harness the unique properties of specific herbs, ensuring maximum potency and efficacy.

Whether you are seeking relief from colds, flu, or other viral illnesses, or simply looking to fortify your immune system and promote overall well-being, you will find a wealth of options within these pages. From immune-boosting elixirs to soothing bath blends, each recipe is designed to support your body's innate ability to heal and thrive.

As you embark on this journey into the world of herbal medicine, may you find inspiration, empowerment, and renewed vitality. May these ancient remedies serve as a beacon of hope and resilience in challenging times, reminding us of the enduring power of nature to heal, nurture, and protect.

With gratitude and reverence for the healing wisdom of generations past, let us embrace the transformative potential of herbal medicine and embark on a path toward greater health and vitality.

Immune-Boosting Elixirs: Herbal Teas, Infusions, and Tonics

Lavender Calmative Drops

On days riddled with anxiety and turmoil, I'd often find solace with granny's lavender concoction, it calmed the nerves and soothed the spirit.

Ingredients: Fresh lavender flowers, alcohol.

Method: Add lavender to a jar and cover with alcohol. Let it steep for 4 weeks, shaking occasionally. Strain.

Usage: 5 drops during moments of stress or before sleep.

Milk Thistle Liver Cleanser

Granny always emphasised the importance of a clean liver. This tincture, she'd say, was her secret to longevity.

Ingredients: Milk thistle seeds, alcohol.
Method: Coarsely grind seeds, add to a jar, cover with alcohol. Infuse for 6 weeks. Strain.
Usage: 10 drops after heavy meals or festivities.

Echinacea Immune Booster

When winter colds loomed, granny would advocate for her echinacea tincture, and we'd emerge from the season unscathed.
Ingredients: Echinacea root, leaves, and flowers, alcohol.
Method: Combine echinacea parts in a jar, cover with alcohol. Store and shake daily for 4 weeks. Strain.
Usage: 5 drops daily during cold and flu season.

Lemon Balm Upliftment Elixir

Lemon balm infused elixir was a staple in granny's home, uplifting the spirit and refreshing the mind on dreary days.

Ingredients: Lemon balm leaves, honey, water.

Method: Steep lemon balm leaves in hot water for 10 minutes. Strain and add honey to taste.

Usage: Sip throughout the day for a mood boost.

Peppermint Digestive Tonic

Granny's peppermint tonic was a remedy for indigestion, bloating, and discomfort after hearty meals, a true digestive saviour.

Ingredients: Peppermint leaves, ginger, honey, water.

Method: Steep peppermint leaves and ginger in hot water for 15 minutes. Strain, add honey to taste.

Usage: Drink after meals to aid digestion.

Astragalus Energy Infusion

For days when fatigue weighed heavy, granny brewed her astragalus infusion, restoring vitality and fortitude.

Ingredients: Astragalus root, honey, water.
Method: Simmer astragalus root in water for 20 minutes. Strain, add honey to taste.
Usage: Sip throughout the day for sustained energy.

Ginger Turmeric Anti-Inflammatory Elixir

Granny's golden elixir of ginger and turmeric was a potent anti-inflammatory, soothing aches and pains with each sip.

Ingredients: Fresh ginger, turmeric, honey, water.
Method: Simmer ginger and turmeric in water for 15 minutes. Strain, add honey to taste.
Usage: Drink daily to reduce inflammation and support overall health.

Elderberry Immune-Boosting Tonic

Elderberry tonic was granny's go-to remedy for warding off colds and flu, strengthening the immune system with each sip.

Ingredients: Dried elderberries, cinnamon, cloves, honey, water.

Method: Simmer elderberries, cinnamon, and cloves in water for 30 minutes. Strain, add honey to taste.

Usage: Take 1 tablespoon daily during cold and flu season.

Rosehip Vitamin C Infusion

Rich in immune-boosting vitamin C, granny's rosehip infusion was a winter essential, warding off illness and keeping us healthy all season long.

Ingredients: Dried rosehips, honey, water.

Method: Steep dried rosehips in hot water for 15 minutes. Strain, add honey to taste.

Usage: Enjoy daily to support immune health.

Licorice Root Soothing Tonic

Granny's licorice root tonic was a balm for sore throats and coughs, soothing inflammation and easing discomfort with its sweet, earthy flavour.

Ingredients: Licorice root, honey, water.
Method: Simmer licorice root in water for 20 minutes. Strain, add honey to taste.
Usage: Drink as needed to alleviate sore throats and coughs.

Potent Tinctures and Extracts: Concentrated Formulas for Viral Defense

Garlic Immune Fortifier

A staple in Granny's arsenal against illness, this pungent tincture was our shield during flu outbreaks and cold seasons.

Ingredients: Fresh garlic cloves, alcohol.
Method: Crush garlic cloves and place them in a jar, covering them with alcohol. Allow to steep for 2 weeks, shaking occasionally. Strain.
Usage: Take 5 drops daily to fortify the immune system

Astragalus Root Vitality Tonic

Known for its immune-boosting properties, astragalus root was a cornerstone of Granny's antiviral remedies, ensuring vitality during times of need.

Ingredients: Dried astragalus root, alcohol.

Method: Place dried astragalus root in a jar and cover with alcohol. Steep for 4 weeks, shaking occasionally. Strain.

Usage: Consume 10 drops daily to support immune health.

Elderberry Syrup for Respiratory Health

During flu season, Granny's elderberry syrup was our go-to remedy for respiratory support, offering relief from coughs and congestion.

Ingredients: Dried elderberries, honey, water.

Method: Simmer dried elderberries in water until reduced by half. Strain and mix with honey. Store in a glass jar.

Usage: Take 1 tablespoon daily during cold and flu season.

Oregano Oil Antiviral Blend

Harnessing the power of oregano's antimicrobial compounds, this potent oil blend was Granny's solution for combating viral infections.

Ingredients: Dried oregano leaves, olive oil.

Method: Infuse dried oregano leaves in olive oil in a jar for 2 weeks. Strain.

Usage: Apply topically to affected areas or ingest 3 drops daily to fight off viruses.

Licorice Root Respiratory Support

With its soothing properties, licorice root was Granny's remedy for respiratory ailments, offering relief from coughs and sore throats.

Ingredients: Dried licorice root, alcohol.

Method: Place dried licorice root in a jar and cover with alcohol. Steep for 3 weeks, shaking occasionally. Strain.

Usage: Take 5 drops daily to support respiratory health.

Thyme Antiviral Infusion

Thyme's potent antiviral properties made it a staple in Granny's herbal apothecary, providing protection against respiratory infections and congestion.

Ingredients: Fresh thyme sprigs, water, honey.

Method: Steep fresh thyme sprigs in hot water for 10 minutes. Strain and sweeten with honey.

Usage: Drink 1 cup daily during cold and flu season.

Goldenseal Root Immune Enhancer

Granny's goldenseal root tincture was our family's safeguard against infections, boosting the immune system and promoting overall health.

Ingredients: Dried goldenseal root, alcohol.

Method: Combine dried goldenseal root and alcohol in a jar. Steep for 4 weeks, shaking occasionally. Strain.

Usage: Take 5 drops daily for immune support.

Sage Antiviral Gargle

For throat infections and mouth sores, Granny's sage gargle provided relief and accelerated healing, thanks to sage's antimicrobial properties.

Ingredients: Fresh sage leaves, water, salt.
Method: Boil fresh sage leaves in water for 10 minutes. Add salt and allow to cool. Gargle several times a day.
Usage: Use as a gargle for sore throats and mouth infections.

Cat's Claw Defence Tonic

Cat's claw, with its immune-stimulating properties, was a cornerstone of Granny's antiviral arsenal, fortifying the body against infections.
Ingredients: Dried cat's claw bark, alcohol.
Method: Place dried cat's claw bark in a jar and cover with alcohol. Steep for 6 weeks, shaking occasionally. Strain.
Usage: Take 10 drops daily to boost immune function.

Peppermint and Ginger Digestive Support

To ease digestive discomfort and boost immunity, Granny's peppermint and ginger tincture provided relief and protection against viral infections.

Ingredients: Fresh peppermint leaves, fresh ginger root, alcohol.

Method: Combine chopped peppermint leaves and ginger root in a jar, covered with alcohol. Steep for 3 weeks, shaking occasionally. Strain.

Usage: Take 5 drops before or after meals to support digestion and immunity.

Herbal Syrups and Oxymels: Soothing Solutions for Respiratory Health

Elderflower Respiratory Syrup

During the peak of cold and flu season, Granny would craft her elderflower syrup, a soothing elixir that provided relief from congestion and respiratory discomfort.

Ingredients: Dried elderflowers, honey, water.

Method: Simmer dried elderflowers in water until reduced by half. Strain and mix with honey. Store in a glass jar.

Usage: Take 1 tablespoon every 4 hours as needed for respiratory relief.

Thyme and Honey Oxymel

With its potent antiviral properties, thyme was a cornerstone of Granny's remedies. Combined with honey, it offered a sweet and effective solution for respiratory infections.

Ingredients: Fresh thyme sprigs, honey, apple cider vinegar.

Method: Combine chopped thyme sprigs with honey and apple cider vinegar in a jar. Let it sit for 2 weeks, shaking occasionally. Strain.

Usage: Take 1 tablespoon daily to support respiratory health.

Licorice Root Soothing Syrup

Licorice root's demulcent properties made it ideal for soothing coughs and sore throats. Granny's licorice syrup was a comforting remedy during times of respiratory distress.

Ingredients: Dried licorice root, honey, water.

Method: Simmer dried licorice root in water until reduced by half. Strain and mix with honey. Store in a glass jar.

Usage: Take 1 teaspoon every 2 hours as needed for throat relief.

Sage and Marshmallow Root Syrup

Granny's sage and marshmallow root syrup was a potent blend for respiratory health, providing relief from coughs and promoting clear breathing.

Ingredients: Fresh sage leaves, dried marshmallow root, honey, water.

Method: Steep sage leaves and marshmallow root in water for 30 minutes. Strain and mix with honey. Store in a glass jar.

Usage: Take 1 tablespoon every 4 hours for cough relief.

Mullein and Plantain Lung Support Syrup

Mullein and plantain, renowned for their respiratory benefits, were combined in Granny's syrup to offer support during bouts of cough and congestion.

Ingredients: Dried mullein leaves, dried plantain leaves, honey, water.

Method: Infuse mullein and plantain leaves in hot water for 20 minutes. Strain and mix with honey. Store in a glass jar.

Usage: Take 1 tablespoon every 3 hours for respiratory support.

Ginger and Turmeric Immune Syrup

Granny's ginger and turmeric syrup was a potent immune booster, providing protection against viral infections and inflammation.

Ingredients: Fresh ginger root, fresh turmeric root, honey, water.

Method: Simmer ginger and turmeric in water until reduced by half. Strain and mix with honey. Store in a glass jar.

Usage: Take 1 tablespoon daily to support immune function.

Rosehip and Elderberry Syrup

Rich in vitamin C and antioxidants, rosehip and elderberry syrup was Granny's go-to remedy for warding off colds and flu.

Ingredients: Dried rosehips, dried elderberries, honey, water.

Method: Simmer rosehips and elderberries in water until reduced by half. Strain and mix with honey. Store in a glass jar.

Usage: Take 1 tablespoon daily during cold and flu season.

Horehound and Coltsfoot Cough Syrup

Granny's horehound and coltsfoot syrup was a traditional remedy for coughs and chest congestion, offering relief and promoting expectoration.

Ingredients: Dried horehound leaves, dried coltsfoot leaves, honey, water.

Method: Steep horehound and coltsfoot leaves in hot water for 20 minutes. Strain and mix with honey. Store in a glass jar.

Usage: Take 1 teaspoon every 3 hours for cough relief.

Hyssop and Thyme Lung Tonic

Hyssop and thyme combined in Granny's syrup to provide respiratory support, soothing coughs and helping to clear congestion.

Ingredients: Fresh hyssop leaves, fresh thyme sprigs, honey, water.

Method: Steep hyssop leaves and thyme sprigs in hot water for 30 minutes. Strain and mix with honey. Store in a glass jar.

Usage: Take 1 tablespoon every 4 hours for lung support.

Plantain and Marshmallow Root Cough Syrup

Granny's plantain and marshmallow root syrup was a gentle yet effective remedy for coughs, providing relief and promoting healing of the respiratory tract.

Ingredients: Dried plantain leaves, dried marshmallow root, honey, water.

Method: Infuse plantain leaves and marshmallow root in hot water for 20 minutes. Strain and mix with honey. Store in a glass jar.

Usage: Take 1 teaspoon every 2 hours for cough relief.

Healing Balms and Salves: Topical Treatments for Skin and Mucosal Infections

Calendula Healing Balm

Granny's calendula balm was a staple in our household, offering relief from skin irritations and promoting wound healing with its soothing properties.

Ingredients: Dried calendula flowers, olive oil, beeswax.

Method: Infuse dried calendula flowers in olive oil using a double boiler method for 4-6 hours. Strain and mix with melted beeswax. Pour into containers to solidify.

Usage: Apply to affected areas as needed for skin healing.

Plantain Salve for Skin Infections

Granny's plantain salve was our go-to remedy for treating cuts, scrapes, and insect bites, thanks to its antimicrobial and anti-inflammatory properties.

Ingredients: Fresh plantain leaves, coconut oil, beeswax.

Method: Infuse fresh plantain leaves in melted coconut oil using a double boiler method for 3-4 hours. Strain and mix with melted beeswax. Pour into containers to solidify.

Usage: Apply topically to affected areas 2-3 times daily for skin infections.

Comfrey Healing Ointment

Granny's comfrey ointment was a potent remedy for promoting tissue repair and relieving pain associated with bruises, sprains, and minor wounds.

Ingredients: Dried comfrey root and leaves, olive oil, beeswax.

Method: Infuse dried comfrey root and leaves in olive oil using a double boiler method for 4-6 hours. Strain and mix with melted beeswax. Pour into containers to solidify.

Usage: Apply to affected areas as needed for tissue healing and pain relief.

Tea Tree and Lavender Antiseptic Salve

Combining the antiseptic properties of tea tree oil with the soothing effects of lavender, Granny's salve was perfect for treating cuts, burns, and skin infections.

Ingredients: Tea tree essential oil, lavender essential oil, coconut oil, beeswax.

Method: Mix melted coconut oil and beeswax, then add tea tree and lavender essential oils. Pour into containers to solidify.

Usage: Apply to clean, dry skin as needed for antiseptic treatment.

Goldenseal Skin Healing Balm

Granny's goldenseal balm was renowned for its powerful antimicrobial and anti-inflammatory properties, making it effective for treating skin infections and promoting healing.

Ingredients: Dried goldenseal root, olive oil, beeswax.

Method: Infuse dried goldenseal root in olive oil using a double boiler method for 4-6 hours. Strain and mix with melted beeswax. Pour into containers to solidify.

Usage: Apply to affected areas 2-3 times daily for skin healing.

Arnica Muscle and Joint Balm

Granny's arnica balm was a trusted remedy for soothing sore muscles and relieving joint pain, providing natural relief from inflammation and stiffness.

Ingredients: Dried arnica flowers, olive oil, beeswax.

Method: Infuse dried arnica flowers in olive oil using a double boiler method for 4-6 hours. Strain and mix with melted beeswax. Pour into containers to solidify.

Usage: Massage onto affected muscles and joints as needed for pain relief.

St. John's Wort Nerve Balm

Granny's St. John's Wort balm was our family's remedy for nerve pain and discomfort, offering relief from conditions such as neuralgia and sciatica.

Ingredients: Dried St. John's Wort flowers, olive oil, beeswax.

Method: Infuse dried St. John's Wort flowers in olive oil using a double boiler method for 4-6 hours. Strain and mix with melted beeswax. Pour into containers to solidify.

Usage: Apply to affected areas for nerve pain relief.

Chamomile and Calendula Soothing Balm

Granny's chamomile and calendula balm was a gentle yet effective remedy for soothing irritated skin, providing relief from conditions such as eczema and dermatitis.

Ingredients: Dried chamomile flowers, dried calendula flowers, olive oil, beeswax.

Method: Infuse dried chamomile and calendula flowers in olive oil using a double boiler method for 4-6 hours. Strain and mix with melted beeswax. Pour into containers to solidify.

Usage: Apply topically to irritated skin as needed for soothing relief.

Yarrow Healing Salve

Granny's yarrow salve was a versatile remedy for promoting wound healing and reducing inflammation, making it useful for treating cuts, scrapes, and bruises.

Ingredients: Dried yarrow flowers and leaves, olive oil, beeswax.

Method: Infuse dried yarrow flowers and leaves in olive oil using a double boiler method for 4-6 hours. Strain and mix with melted beeswax. Pour into containers to solidify.

Usage: Apply to clean, dry skin as needed for wound healing.

Garlic and Thyme Antimicrobial Balm

Granny's garlic and thyme balm was a potent antimicrobial blend, ideal for treating fungal infections, cold sores, and other skin ailments.

Ingredients: Fresh garlic cloves, fresh thyme sprigs, olive oil, beeswax.

Method: Infuse chopped garlic cloves and thyme sprigs in olive oil using a double boiler method for 4-6 hours. Strain and mix with melted beeswax. Pour into containers **to solidify.**

Usage: Apply to affected areas 2-3 times daily for antimicrobial treatment.

Culinary Creations for Immune Support: Incorporating Antiviral Herbs into Everyday Cooking

Rosemary Infused Olive Oil

Granny's rosemary-infused olive oil was a staple in our kitchen, adding not just flavour but also antiviral properties to our dishes.

Ingredients: Fresh rosemary sprigs, extra virgin olive oil.

Method: Place rosemary sprigs in a glass jar and cover completely with olive oil. Let it infuse for 2 weeks in a cool, dark place, shaking occasionally. Strain before use.

Usage: Use in salad dressings, marinades, or drizzle over roasted vegetables for added flavour and immune support.

Thyme and Garlic Roasted Chicken

Granny's thyme and garlic roasted chicken wasn't just a hearty meal but also a powerful immune-boosting dish, thanks to the antiviral properties of thyme and garlic.

Ingredients: Whole chicken, fresh thyme sprigs, garlic cloves, olive oil, salt, pepper.

Method: Rub the chicken with olive oil, minced garlic, chopped thyme, salt, and pepper. Roast in the oven until golden brown and cooked through.

Usage: Serve as a main dish for a nourishing meal that supports immune health.

Basil Pesto Pasta

Granny's basil pesto pasta was a family favourite, not just for its delicious taste but also for the antiviral properties of basil, garlic, and olive oil.

Ingredients: Fresh basil leaves, garlic cloves, pine nuts, Parmesan cheese, extra virgin olive oil, salt, pepper.

Method: Blend basil leaves, garlic, pine nuts, and Parmesan cheese in a food processor. Gradually add olive oil until smooth. Season with salt and pepper. Toss with cooked pasta.

Usage: Enjoy as a flavorful and immune-supporting pasta dish.

Ginger Turmeric Tea

Granny's ginger turmeric tea was a comforting beverage during cold seasons, providing warmth and immune-boosting properties.

Ingredients: Fresh ginger root, fresh turmeric root, lemon, honey.

Method: Grate ginger and turmeric into a pot of boiling water. Simmer for 10-15 minutes. Strain and add lemon juice and honey to taste.

Usage: Sip on this soothing tea to support immune function and ward off viral infections.

Oregano Lemon Chicken Soup

Granny's oregano lemon chicken soup was a nourishing bowl of comfort, enriched with the antiviral properties of oregano and the immune-boosting benefits of lemon.

Ingredients: Chicken broth, cooked chicken, carrots, celery, onion, garlic, fresh oregano, lemon juice, salt, pepper.

Method: Simmer chicken broth with vegetables, garlic, and oregano until tender. Add cooked chicken and lemon juice. Season with salt and pepper.

Usage: Enjoy a bowl of this hearty soup to fortify the immune system and combat viral infections.

Sage and Honey Roasted Sweet Potatoes

Granny's sage and honey roasted sweet potatoes were not only a delicious side dish but also a source of immune-supporting antioxidants from sage and honey.

Ingredients: Sweet potatoes, fresh sage leaves, honey, olive oil, salt, pepper.

Method: Toss sweet potato chunks with chopped sage leaves, honey, olive oil, salt, and pepper. Roast until caramelised and tender.

Usage: Serve as a flavorful accompaniment to any meal for a boost of antiviral properties.

Cinnamon Ginger Golden Milk

Granny's cinnamon ginger golden milk was a soothing bedtime drink, rich in immune-boosting spices like cinnamon and ginger.

Ingredients: Turmeric powder, cinnamon powder, ginger powder, black pepper, honey, milk.

Method: Warm milk in a saucepan and whisk in turmeric, cinnamon, ginger, black pepper, and honey. Simmer for a few minutes until fragrant.

Usage: Enjoy a cup of this comforting golden milk before bedtime for its antiviral and immune-supporting benefits.

Parsley Walnut Pesto

Granny's parsley walnut pesto was a vibrant and nutritious spread, packed with the antiviral properties of parsley and the omega-3 fatty acids from walnuts.

Ingredients: Fresh parsley leaves, walnuts, garlic cloves, Parmesan cheese, extra virgin olive oil, salt, pepper.

Method: Blend parsley, walnuts, garlic, and Parmesan cheese in a food processor. Gradually add olive oil until smooth. Season with salt and pepper.

Usage: Spread on toast, sandwiches, or use as a dip for vegetables for a flavorful and immune-boosting snack.

Garlic Lemon Broccoli Stir-Fry

Granny's garlic lemon broccoli stir-fry was a quick and healthy dish, enhanced with the antiviral properties of garlic and the immune-boosting benefits of lemon.

Ingredients: Broccoli florets, garlic cloves, lemon zest, soy sauce, olive oil, salt, pepper.

Method: Stir-fry broccoli in olive oil with minced garlic until tender. Add lemon zest, soy sauce, salt, and pepper to taste.

Usage: Serve as a nutritious side dish or add protein for a complete meal that supports immune health.

Chive and Dill Yogurt Dip

Granny's chive and dill yoghourt dip was a refreshing and immune-boosting accompaniment to vegetable crudités or whole-grain crackers.

Ingredients: Greek yoghourt, fresh chives, fresh dill, lemon juice, salt, pepper.

Method: Mix Greek yoghourt with chopped chives, dill, lemon juice, salt, and pepper until well combined.

Usage: Serve as a healthy dip for a snack or appetiser, providing antiviral properties from chives and dill.

Herbal Antiviral Baths and Steams

Eucalyptus Steam Inhalation

Granny's eucalyptus steam inhalation was a revitalising experience, clearing congested sinuses and providing relief from respiratory ailments.

Ingredients: Fresh eucalyptus leaves, boiling water.

Method: Place eucalyptus leaves in a bowl and cover with boiling water. Lean over the bowl with a towel over your head to trap the steam. Inhale deeply for 5-10 minutes.

Usage: Enjoy this steam inhalation 2-3 times a day to alleviate symptoms of viral infections such as colds or sinusitis.

Peppermint Lavender Bath Salts

Granny's peppermint lavender bath salts were a luxurious treat, offering relaxation and immune support with every soak.

Ingredients: Epsom salt, baking soda, dried peppermint leaves, lavender essential oil.

Method: Mix Epsom salt and baking soda in a bowl. Add dried peppermint leaves and a few drops of lavender essential oil. Stir well and store in a jar.

Usage: Add a handful of bath salts to warm bathwater and soak for 20 minutes to unwind and boost immune function.

Rosemary Thyme Herbal Bath

Granny's rosemary thyme herbal bath was a fragrant and invigorating ritual, promoting circulation and fortifying the body against viral infections.

Ingredients: Fresh rosemary sprigs, fresh thyme sprigs, boiling water.

Method: Tie rosemary and thyme sprigs together and steep in a pot of boiling water for 30 minutes. Strain and pour into a warm bath.

Usage: Relax in the herbal-infused bathwater for 20-30 minutes to soothe muscles and support immune health.

Ginger Chamomile Foot Soak

Granny's ginger chamomile foot soak was a rejuvenating experience, relieving fatigue and boosting immunity through the feet's reflex points.

Ingredients: Fresh ginger root, dried chamomile flowers, warm water.

Method: Grate fresh ginger into a basin of warm water and add dried chamomile flowers. Soak feet for 20-30 minutes.

Usage: Enjoy this foot soak before bedtime to promote relaxation and enhance immune function.

Lemon Verbena Herbal Bath Tea

Granny's lemon verbena herbal bath tea was a fragrant and uplifting addition to bath time, offering antiviral properties and a refreshing aroma.

Ingredients: Dried lemon verbena leaves, muslin bag or tea infuser.

Method: Fill a muslin bag or tea infuser with dried lemon verbena leaves and hang under the faucet as the bath fills. Allow the water to infuse with the herbal goodness.

Usage: Take a leisurely bath, allowing the lemon verbena aroma to uplift your spirits and support immune health.

Thyme Rose Petal Bath Soak

Granny's thyme rose petal bath soak was a luxurious indulgence, combining the antiviral properties of thyme with the soothing fragrance of rose petals.

Ingredients: Fresh thyme sprigs, dried rose petals, Epsom salt, warm water.

Method: Tie thyme sprigs and dried rose petals together in a muslin cloth. Place in a bathtub filled with warm water and add Epsom salt.

Usage: Soak in the bath for 20-30 minutes, allowing the herbal blend to promote relaxation and immune support.

Lavender Echinacea Bath Bomb

Granny's lavender echinacea bath bomb was a fizzy delight, infusing the bathwater with calming lavender and immune-boosting echinacea.

Ingredients: Baking soda, citric acid, cornstarch, dried lavender flowers, dried echinacea leaves, lavender essential oil, witch hazel.

Method: Mix baking soda, citric acid, and cornstarch in a bowl. Add dried lavender flowers, dried echinacea leaves, and lavender essential oil. Spritz with witch hazel until the mixture holds its shape. Press into moulds and let dry.

Usage: Drop one bath bomb into warm bathwater and watch it fizz while releasing its herbal goodness.

Peppermint Tea Tree Foot Spray

Granny's peppermint tea tree foot spray was a refreshing and antiviral solution for tired feet, providing a cooling sensation and protection against infections.

Ingredients: Peppermint essential oil, tea tree essential oil, witch hazel, distilled water.

Method: Mix peppermint and tea tree essential oils with witch hazel and distilled water in a spray bottle. Shake well before each use.

Usage: Spray onto clean feet and massage gently for a cooling and invigorating experience that supports immune health.

Rosemary Sage Bath Salt Scrub

Granny's rosemary sage bath salt scrub was a rejuvenating exfoliant, combining the antiviral properties of rosemary and sage with the cleansing action of salt.

Ingredients: Epsom salt, sea salt, olive oil, fresh rosemary leaves, fresh sage leaves.

Method: Mix Epsom salt, sea salt, and olive oil in a bowl. Add chopped rosemary and sage leaves. Scrub onto damp skin in the shower, then rinse off.

Usage: Use once or twice a week to exfoliate and nourish the skin while enjoying the immune-boosting benefits of herbs.

Chamomile Lavender Bath Oil

Granny's chamomile lavender bath oil was a luxurious addition to bath time, promoting relaxation and immune support with its soothing fragrance.

Ingredients: Chamomile essential oil, lavender essential oil, carrier oil (such as almond or jojoba).

Method: Mix chamomile and lavender essential oils with a carrier oil in a glass bottle. Shake well before each use.

Usage: Add a few drops of bath oil to warm bathwater and soak for 20 minutes to calm the mind and strengthen the immune system.

Conclusion: Empowering Your Journey with Herbal Antivirals

As we reach the culmination of our exploration into the world of herbal antivirals, it's essential to reflect on the transformative power that lies within the embrace of nature's wisdom. Throughout this journey, we've delved deep into the healing properties of plants, discovering their remarkable ability to combat viral infections and bolster our immune systems. From ancient remedies passed down through generations to modern scientific discoveries, we've witnessed the profound impact that herbal medicine can have on our health and well-being.

But beyond the mere efficacy of herbal antivirals lies a deeper truth—a truth that speaks to the interconnectedness of all life and the inherent wisdom of the natural world. In our quest for health and vitality, we often find ourselves seeking solutions outside of ourselves, relying on synthetic medications and external interventions to heal our ailments. Yet, as we've discovered, the true power to heal lies within the very fabric of our being, waiting to be awakened and nurtured by the gifts of the earth.

In embracing herbal antivirals, we are not merely treating symptoms or suppressing illness; we are reclaiming our innate ability to heal and thrive. We are reconnecting with the wisdom of our ancestors, who understood the healing power of plants long before modern medicine existed. We are acknowledging our place within the intricate web of life, recognizing that our health is intimately intertwined with the health of the planet.

As we move forward on our journey, let us heed the call to action that herbal antivirals present. Let us cultivate a deeper relationship with the natural world, honouring and respecting the plants that sustain us. Let us embrace a holistic approach to health, recognizing that true wellness encompasses not only the absence of disease but the presence of vitality and balance in body, mind, and spirit.

In doing so, we empower ourselves to take control of our health and well-being, to become active participants in our own healing journey. We become stewards of the earth, protecting and preserving the precious resources that sustain life. And we become agents of change, advocating for a future where herbal medicine is recognized and respected as a cornerstone of health care.

As we close this chapter and embark on the next phase of our journey, let us carry with us the knowledge, wisdom, and inspiration that herbal antivirals provide. Let us embrace the healing power of nature and the limitless potential that resides within each of us. And let us step boldly into the future, empowered by the gifts of the earth and guided by the wisdom of generations past.

The time to embrace herbal antivirals is now. Together, let us embark on this journey of healing, empowerment, and transformation, and let us create a world where health and vitality are accessible to all.